MOVIES, MUSIC AND MEMORY

Emerald Studies in the Humanities, Ageing and Later Life

Series Editor

Kate de Medeiros, Miami University, USA

Emerald Studies in the Humanities, Ageing and Later Life responds to the growing need for scholarship focused on age, identity and meaning in late life in a time of unprecedented longevity. For the first time in human history, there are more people in the world aged 60 years and over than under age five. In response, empirical gerontological research on how and why we age has seen exponential growth. An unintended consequence of this growth, however, has been an increasing chasm between the need to study age through generalizable data – the "objective" – and the importance of understanding the human experience of growing old.

Emerald Studies in the Humanities, Ageing and Later Life bridges this gap. The series creates a more intellectually diversified gerontology through the perspective of the humanities as well as other interpretive, non-empirical approaches that draw from humanities scholarship. Publishing monographs, edited collections and short-form Emerald Points volumes, the series represents the most cutting-edge research in the areas of humanistic gerontology and ageing.

Editorial Board

MOVIES, MUSIC AND MEMORY

Tools for Wellbeing in Later Life

Emerald Studies in the Humanities, Ageing and Later Life

EDITED BY

JULIA HALLAM
University of Liverpool, UK

LISA SHAW
University of Liverpool, UK

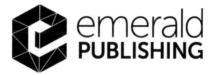

United Kingdom – North America – Japan – India
Malaysia – China

Emerald Publishing Limited
Howard House, Wagon Lane, Bingley BD16 1WA, UK

First edition 2020

British Library Cataloguing in Publication Data
A catalogue record for this book is available from the British Library

ISBN: 978-1-83909-202-2 (Print)
ISBN: 978-1-83909-199-5 (Online)
ISBN: 978-1-83909-201-5 (Epub)

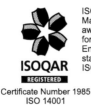

ISOQAR certified
Management System,
awarded to Emerald
for adherence to
Environmental
standard
ISO 14001:2004.

Certificate Number 1985
ISO 14001

INVESTOR IN PEOPLE

For our parents

CONTENTS

LIST OF FIGURES

ABOUT THE CONTRIBUTORS

Julia Hallam is Professor Emerita in the Department of Communication and Media, School of the Arts, University of Liverpool. She has written widely on issues of gender, representation and aesthetics in film and media and on women as creators and producers of film and television. More recently, she led three AHRC-funded projects on film, memory and urban space, working with amateur and independent filmmakers, the North West Film Archive and the British Film Institute. She has curated exhibitions for the National Museum of Medicine, Washington DC, and the Museum of Liverpool. In an earlier life, she trained as a nurse and health visitor and led the Liverpool arm of the Neighbourhood Health Project (1977–1979), one of the first projects in the UK to employ community health workers to co-ordinate new initiatives on health and social care issues.

Lisa Shaw is Professor of Brazilian Studies in the Department of Modern Languages and Cultures at the University of Liverpool. Her research interests are Brazilian cultural history, with an emphasis on twentieth-century popular music, theatre and film, and in particular from a transnational perspective. She has written books on the social history of Brazilian samba music, the film star Carmen Miranda and popular Brazilian cinema from the 1940s and 1950s. She leads the *Cinema,*

Memory and Wellbeing impact project, which explores the use of music and film as reminiscence tools to improve the emotional wellbeing of the older population, including those living with a dementia diagnosis, and involves outreach initiatives on Merseyside, UK, and in the states of Rio de Janeiro and São Paulo, Brazil.

Dr Jacqueline Waldock is a researcher at the University of Liverpool. She previously studied Music at Lancaster University and went on to complete a doctorate at the University of Liverpool in Musicology and Composition. Her research focusses on sounds of everyday life, listening cultures and soundscape composition as an ethnographic tool. Selected publications include: Waldock, J. (2016). Hearing urban change. In L. Black & M. Bull (Eds.), *Auditory cultural reader* (2nd revised edition). Bloomsbury and Waldock, J. (2016). Crossing the boundaries: Community composition and sensory ethnography. *Senses and Society*, *11*(1), 60–67.

Sara Cohen is a Professor at the University of Liverpool where she holds the James and Constance Alsop Chair in Music and is Director of the Institute of Popular Music. She has a DPhil in Social Anthropology from Oxford University and is author of *Rock Culture in Liverpool* (1991) and *Decline, Renewal and the City in Popular Music Culture* (2007), co-author of *Harmonious Relations* (1994) and *Liverpool's Musical Landscapes* (2018) and co-editor of *Sites of Popular Music Heritage* (2014). She has specialized in interdisciplinary research on popular music, with a particular interest in ethnographic approaches and research on place, heritage, memory and ageing.

Helena Culshaw is an independent occupational therapist and former chair and vice-chair of the Royal College of Occupational Therapists. Helena has previously managed services in the NHS in both hospital and community services including mental health.

Dr Clarissa Giebel is a dementia care researcher, based at the University of Liverpool at the National Institute for Health Research ARC NWC (Applied Research Collaboration North West Coast). Her main research focus is on enabling people with dementia to live independently for longer in the community, thereby addressing potential health inequalities that might affect access to the right care at the right time. She is leading on a number of projects in this field, and works closely with the Netherlands, Australia, Colombia and Chile in addressing health inequalities on a global level. Public involvement is a key component of all her work, and she is actively working with people living with dementia and family carers in all her projects. She conducts independent research funded by the NIHR ARC NWC, and the views expressed in this book are her own, not necessarily those of the National Institute for Health Research or the Department of Health and Social Care.

Ros Jennings is Professor of Ageing, Culture and Media and Co-Director of the Women, Ageing and Media (WAM) Research Centre, University of Gloucestershire.

PREFACE

HELENA CULSHAW*

My involvement with this project has been as a catalyst between the contributing authors and practitioner occupational therapists in the North West of England and more specifically those working with dementia patients in the Mersey Care NHS Foundation Trust. When I met with Professor Lisa Shaw and Dr Jacqueline Waldock they told me about the project with older people and the development of the *Cinema, Memory and Wellbeing* toolkit. I could immediately see the potential for their use within Occupational Therapy services for older people and those living with dementia as part of a range of interventions using meaningful activity to trigger memories and promote wellbeing.

This is a well-researched project involving activities suitable for use within any health interventions by therapists who are always keen to investigate the use of occupation-focussed activities that are evidence-based and that will assist their users in being able to participate as they choose. I was particularly struck by the two creative workshops that the contributors held on Merseyside, where they enabled the

---

participants, along with their therapists and carers, to use a variety of crafting techniques to make decorative objects related to the film prior to their viewing it. This created great opportunities for engaging individuals, prompting childhood memories and promoting interaction between the participants. The potential I had seen at the first meeting had come to fruition.

The joy of this book and toolkit is that it can be used to very good effect by staff and carers in nursing and care homes and day centres for older people, as it provides good guidance and tips as well as demonstrating how to use equipment and resources that are easily available every day. Occupational therapists have long used creative activities as meaningful occupation within their interventions with service users, including older people. The outcome of this project is complementary to occupational therapy, and I would recommend its usefulness within specific interventions in health and care settings by occupational therapists seeking to extend the range of opportunities for service users.

Reminiscence work with older people and people living with dementia is constantly moving forwards. As the age profile changes, so does the era of the movies and the music that can be profitably used in reminiscence work. This project shows that these principles and the toolkit could be applied to re-connect people with memories from the eras of Carmen Miranda or Madonna, of Gershwin or Gary Barlow.

INTRODUCTION: MAPPING THE TERRAIN – FILM AND MUSIC IN THIRD-AGE CARE

Julia Hallam, Lisa Shaw and Jacqueline Waldock

AGEING AND DEMENTIA: THE UK AND GLOBAL CONTEXTS

The ageing population and the increase in those living with a dementia diagnosis present a major societal challenge and threat to the systems and institutions that maintain the wellbeing and welfare of older members of modernized societies. The number of people in England and Wales aged over 65 years will increase by roughly 19.4% by 2025. Notably, the number of people in the UK aged over 85 years is likely to double in the next 25 years. These projections are supported by recent high-profile reports, including one in *Lancet Public Health*, urging the government 'to give urgent consideration to options for more cost-effective health and social care provision in all its forms', and emphasizing that 'informal and home care require stronger policy support' (Castillo et al., 2017, p. 312). As we get older in life, the loss of partners and friends to share our memories with, combined with the increasing chance of health and mobility issues, can cause loneliness, anxiety and distress. Coupled with this is the fact that people are generally living longer, families are more mobile and adult children sometimes live far away from their ageing parents. In the UK, increased life expectancy is already giving rise to a crisis in care that can leave older people unsupported in their homes, and unable to afford community-based or residential care. Attempts to help alleviate loneliness and its associated emotional diffi-culties by providing activities that bring people together, be it in community day-care facilities or the communal areas of retirement and nursing homes, have mushroomed in recent years. Despite funding challenges, charities, social enterprise initiatives and public organizations are finding ways to enable care workers, carers and volunteers to become involved in providing a wide range of activities for older people, many of them based on various forms of reminis-cence and memory work. Participation in these activities, often drawing on artefacts and images from the past, has been shown to demonstrably enhance the wellbeing of those taking part, both the carers and the cared for.

Caring for a growing population of older people, and particularly those living with dementia-related cognitive impairment, is a major global health and development challenge; as well as impacting on the lives of those with a dementia diagnosis, it is now widely recognized that care-givers and family members need both emotional and prac-tical support. This threat to welfare is particularly acute in developing countries and emerging economies like Brazil, whose senior population is predicted to exceed 32 million by 2025 (US Census Bureau), where the vast majority of people aged 60 years and over (73%) and of those aged 80 years and over (80%) are currently dependent on the poorly funded, increasingly precarious, state health-care system (SUS), and where there are over a million people living with a dementia diagnosis (although it is widely recognized that under-diagnosis of dementia is high in low- and middle-income countries). It is estimated that there is only one geriatrician per 22,000 older people in Brazil, and that large geographical areas have virtually non-existent geriatric coverage (Garcez-Lemme & Deckers Lemme, 2014, p. 3). Only 1% of the growing ageing population of this country, the largest nation in South America, with a population of over 200 million people, live in long-term care homes, and frequently people with dementia live with their families, with some support from civil or religious organizations, and home visits from the *Programa Saúde da Família* (PSF – Family Health Programme). As Garcez-Lemme and Deckers-Lemme write: 'The problem of the elderly in Brazil requires solutions applicable to a rapidly growing population, with […] very limited financial resources and scant family support. Solutions must be simple, easily applicable, with a good cost-benefit relationship' (2014, p. 3).

Care for people living with dementia and for the family members who care for them differs greatly from one national context to another. As Clarissa Giebel, one of the contributors to this book, has noted: 'Some European countries have only recently implemented national dementia strategies, and structures and content of services vary greatly, which may suggest that countries need to address issues of independence and well-being in dementia in the light of these' (Giebel et al., 2014). The Right Time Place Care study has explored dementia care provision at the transition point from home residence to living in a care home, examining and comparing the factors that affect care home admission and costs for people living with dementia across the UK, Germany, the Netherlands, Spain, Estonia, Sweden, France and Finland (Verbeek et al., 2012). One of the many symptoms which requires support in dementia care

are difficulties with basic activities such as getting dressed, as well as more complex activities, such as dealing with personal medication and finance management, or even making a hot drink. People with dementia in its earliest stages may lose the ability to initiate and perform these more complex activities, along with other manifestations of cognitive deterioration, but are still able to carry out the more basic tasks, such as washing themselves and dressing, until the disease is more advanced. Clarissa Giebel led a study that looked at these symptoms across the eight countries listed above, concluding, for example, that the ability to bathe and dress oneself deteriorates earlier than the ability to feed oneself (Giebel et al., 2014). She and her research team found that not being able to engage in certain daily activities can affect the quality of life of the person living with dementia, but that these effects vary from country to country, with quality of life only being linked to everyday task performance in the early stages of dementia in some countries, such as Estonia. Quality of life and quality of care in general were found to be highest in the UK and Sweden, and lowest in Estonia and Spain (Beerens et al., 2014). This clearly highlights that within Europe, possibly due to cultural factors as well as system variations in care provision, people with dementia receive different levels of care. These variations can also lead to differences in predictors of care home access across Europe. Whilst caregiver burden and difficulties in engaging with activities of daily living are the main predictors of care home admission relating to dementia across Europe, there are strong country variations. In Germany, for example, depressive symptoms predicted care home admission, whereas this was not the case for France or the Netherlands (Verbeek et al., 2015).

There is clearly a great deal to be done in terms of sharing learning and best practice between different countries, even within developed Europe, and an even more urgent need to disseminate expertise and practical applications of research findings to middle- and low-income countries. It is our hope that, having already translated our best-practice toolkit into Portuguese, we can in the future make it available in a range of other languages, tailored to the specificities of other national contexts, including parts of the developing world.

SOCIAL PRESCRIBING, THE ARTS AND CO-PRODUCTION

One contribution to addressing the crisis in social care in the UK is the development of so-called social prescribing, defined by the CentreForum Mental Health Commission in 2014 as 'a mechanism for linking patients with non-medical sources of support within the community' (CentreForum, online). According to the Kings Fund, social prescribing is designed to enable general practitioners (GPs), nurses and other primary care professionals, such as occupational therapists (OTs), to refer people to a range of local, non-clinical services. These can be activities such as arts and crafts, dance or gardening, wellbeing sessions (meditation, mindfulness, yoga and tai chi, for example) and other services such as diet advice and befriending (The Kings Fund, 2017, online). Social prescribing focusses on prevention of illness and the promotion of wellness rather than treatment, and reflects a paradigm shift that has taken place in our understanding of health and health care in the UK and beyond, one that, as Lisa discovered, has also gathered momentum in Brazil. Flagship arts-based social prescribing projects that have brought universities into close partnership with cultural institutions in the UK include the Arts and Humanities

Research Council (AHRC)-funded Museums on Prescription programme, involving University College London and Canterbury Christ Church University (from which the 'wellbeing umbrellas' measures we tried out in one of our projects in Brazil, discussed in Chapter 3, were adapted). There was initially a certain reluctance among GPs to embrace the concept of social prescribing, a reluctance that appears to be less obvious among nursing staff and link workers; as Lisa and Jacky heard at a regional conference of OTs in 2019, there is still work to be done in reassuring health professionals of the benefits of social prescribing and, perhaps more importantly, how it can be embraced to improve their own working lives.

Social prescribing aims to provide a holistic approach to health care by helping people to take more control of their personal health needs. It recognizes that many of the aspects involved in maintaining a healthy lifestyle are determined by a range of economic, social and environmental factors that are beyond the control of any single individual. It is designed to help people with a wide range of social, emotional and/or practical needs, including those with mild or long-term mental health issues and those who are socially isolated. In 2014 the creation of an All-Party Parliamentary Group on Arts, Health and Wellbeing further evidenced the emphasis at national level of the promotion of wellness via arts-based interventions and has strengthened arguments for their adequate funding (culturehealthandwellbeing.org.uk). Furthermore, in 2018 the UK Government's Health and Wellbeing Fund awarded £4.5 million to 23 social prescribing projects, which led to funding for social prescribing link workers based within NHS trusts to be allocated for the first time in 2019.

Many social prescribing activities are run locally by voluntary groups and charitable organizations that have a particular focus on improving mental health and wellbeing. The standard model is for interventions to be run over a 10-week period and evaluated by end-of-project interviews with participants and facilitators. This 10-week referral model has its limitations, and generally speaking the longer-term benefits of such interventions require further research. A notable exception of a long-term project with a strong research dimension is the work carried out by The Reader, a global organization based in Liverpool, which has produced impressive results when using shared reading activities with people living with dementia, amongst many other groups. As the organization's website states in relation to the conclusions of a six-month study funded by the Headley Trust:

> *the literature-based intervention provided by* Shared Reading *produces a significant reduction in dementia symptoms and benefits the quality of life of both the residents and staff carers. The quantitative and qualitative research also found that short- and long-term memory was positively influenced, listening skills were improved and the provision of activity by an external organisation enhanced patient care* (Gallagher, 2017)

There is a growing body of evidence of the benefits of all forms of arts-based or cultural activity for older adults and those living with dementia, stemming from research conducted across a wide range of disciplines associated with the wellbeing and care of these groups in society, such as psychology, gerontology, psychiatry and the associated professions of nursing and occupational therapy. Research from various perspectives has shown that all of these activities create positive effects in terms of improved mood and cognitive ability (see, for example, Young, Camic, & Tischler, 2016).

These positive effects can be further enhanced by involving participants in the planning and elaboration of the activities in question, what the academic literature refers to as co-design, co-curation or co-production. As we recommend in the toolkit that we designed based on the various pilot projects discussed in this book (downloadable from Emerald's website) – which was created by using a user-centred approach – the involvement of stakeholders in the preparation and design of wellbeing interventions using music and/or film adds a further therapeutic benefit. For those living with dementia, involvement in creative activities has proved to be particularly powerful. Furthermore, arts-based interventions, where the emphasis is taken away from formal education and fact-based learning, has been shown to be a very effective way of assisting the dementia care workforce (Windle et al., 2019). Arts-based activities, like the creative workshops organized at the Plaza Community Cinema on Merseyside as part of the 'Cinema, Memory and Wellbeing Festival' discussed in Chapter 3, optimize and celebrate the abilities that people with dementia still have, providing more of a 'level playing field' that allows them to engage, express themselves and connect with other people.

The projects that we have piloted in the UK and Brazil are a contribution to a growing international body of knowledge that demonstrates that various forms of arts-based or culturally focussed activities make a positive difference to the emotional wellbeing of senior members of society, particularly those living alone or in institutions, and those living with a dementia diagnosis. A dementia study published in the health journal *PLOS Medicine* concluded: 'relatively simple things, if implemented robustly, can actually make a real difference to people's quality of life', particularly if this involves interaction and learning about people's interests and abilities, and can 'help reduce costs, both in care homes and the wider social care system' (Therrien, 2018). This conclusion is an extremely important one and sums up the rationale for all the projects we discuss in this book.

WELLBEING AND OUR MOTIVATIONS

Driving all the projects we discuss in this book is the belief that sharing reminiscences triggered by popular films and popular music, and more specifically film stars, musical performers and images of local places, alongside personal memories of cinema-going, dancing and going to music venues, can create feelings of wellbeing among older people. We begin by looking at a range of projects that have inspired us and the relevant underpinning research. All the projects that we discuss, 'take people out of themselves', people who may otherwise remain isolated in their own internal worlds; by creating opportunities for sharing past experiences, these initiatives enhance the participants' quality of life by re-establishing a sense of personhood in the present. Before talking about some of the specific projects that have informed our own research and practice, however, it is worth pausing to consider what exactly we mean when we talk about wellbeing.

The UK Care Act 2014 (online) defines wellbeing as a broad concept that relates to the following areas in particular:

- Personal dignity (including treatment of the individual with respect)

- Physical and mental health and emotional wellbeing

- Protection from abuse and neglect

- Control by the individual over their day-to-day life (including over care and support provided and the way they are provided)

- Participation in work, education, training or recreation

- Social and economic wellbeing

- Domestic, family and personal domains

- Suitability of living accommodation

- The individual's contribution to society

The first two of these areas – 'personal dignity' and 'physical and mental health and emotional wellbeing' – fall firmly within the remit of the work that we discuss in this book. The evaluation of our pilot projects, explored in the following chapters, hinges on this definition of wellbeing. With this definition in mind, and considering the variety of settings and contexts in which older people can find themselves, such as attending day-care centres or living in nursing homes, helping people to feel good about themselves seems to be of vital importance to their mental health. Amongst older people, depression and anxiety are often a result of loneliness, of struggling to meet the challenges of everyday life with no one to help. If people are anxious and depressed, their ability to meet these challenges in situations where they may have less control over their daily lives than they have been accustomed to in the past is compromised. This is increasingly recognized by doctors and others who care for older people; social pre-scribing, as discussed above, advocates various kinds of activities rather than relying on drug therapy alone as a way of altering mood and enhancing emotional wellbeing.

In this book, we outline four associated, interlinked and developing projects that endeavour to make academic research in the arts and humanities of practical relevance for all kinds of care contexts, and to make related resources both accessible and entertaining for older people. We will discuss the projects in the order in which they have taken place, illustrating how the previous experiences shaped the evolution of our approach and methodology. The projects have developed organically over several years, driven by the energy and enthusiasm of our project leader Lisa Shaw, who saw the care available to her own father after his dementia diagnosis as presenting a real-life challenge that her research could help to address. We will discuss the ways in which we set about measuring improvements in emotional wellbeing, as experienced by both the cared for and those doing the caring, in more depth in Chapters 1 and 3. For our purposes here, we want to point out that all the projects we have carried out were premised on the definition of wellbeing outlined above: they all seek, in various ways, to enhance the quality of life of older people. We will now look at some of the work that has, in various ways, encouraged us to develop our own projects. We will also review some of the academic research that seeks to measure and evaluate the effects of memory and reminiscence work and participatory arts activities on older people.

INSPIRATIONAL REMINISCENCE PROJECTS AND TOOLS

Group reminiscence improved psychological wellbeing of institutionalised elders by decreasing depression and increasing self-esteem, life satisfaction and quality of life (Gaggioli et al., 2014 in Tamura-Lis, 2017, pp. 154–155)

Nowadays many care workers, nurses and others working with older people are using various forms of 'life story' and reminiscence therapy to improve the wellbeing of people attending day centres, and those living in residential care homes and nursing homes, as well as people in long-term hospital care. The 8th edition of *Mosby's Medical Dictionary* (2009) defines reminiscence therapy as a psychotherapeutic technique in which self-esteem and personal satisfaction are restored, particularly in older people, by encouraging patients to review past experiences of a pleasant nature (cited in Latha et al., 2014, p. 1). At its most basic, reminiscence encourages the sharing of memories, often encouraged by a relative, volunteer or professional carer through the use of questions and various kinds of prompts such as artefacts from the past.

The first project we would like to discuss has been a source of particular inspiration and support for our reminiscence-centred work. The *House of Memories* initiative was developed by National Museums Liverpool (NML) from their Generations Apart reminiscence programme (2000), which used so-called 'memory boxes' to prompt remembering. The Generations Apart programme enabled carers and volunteers to borrow specially designed 'memory boxes' containing objects from the Museum's collections – ranging from household objects to work tools, from old cinema tickets and theatre play bills to clothes and popular collectors' items such as cigarette cards or postcards – to stimulate reminiscences and discussion about past times, sometimes with individuals and often in group settings. The success of the 'memory boxes' led NML to develop the award-winning *House of Memories* dementia awareness programme, which 'provides health, social care, housing professionals and family carers with unique and innovative training, and resources inspired by museum collections, to help people to live well with dementia.' (House of Memories, online). 'Memory suitcases' can still be borrowed from the museums, and a free *My House of Memories* app has been developed to facilitate off-site participation and wider engagement. The programme has since been rolled out across a range of museums at national level, and its effectiveness is internationally recognized. The *My House of Memories* app is designed for carers to use with individuals; a wide range of digitized images, arranged by theme, such as school, work and leisure, are available to arrange and save in digital memory trees, memory boxes and timelines. The app can also store personal memories of precious past times, perhaps shared with a partner who has become an individual's carer.

For professional carers working with people with memory loss and/or a dementia diagnosis, creating a personal digital 'life story' is becoming an increasingly popular tool. A similar initiative to the *My House of Memories* app is the *Memory Box Network* charity's on-line system of support, provided by Dundee city council, that uses personal photos and self-chosen images to stimulate memory and reminiscence amongst those who are isolated and living alone, as well as people living with a dementia diagnosis and their carers (dundeecity.gov.uk). Group projects are increasingly common; we have selected just a few of the many projects that feature reminiscence workshops, which demonstrate the range and variety of venues and locations in which they take place. In Lancashire, for example, a not-for-profit community-interest company, *My Colourful Memories*, provides therapeutic arts workshops in libraries, care homes, schools and other communal spaces, with the aim of improving cognitive health. The themes of two of these workshops – 'Music and Memory' and 'Movie Memories' – chime with our own interests and feature light-hearted quizzes to stimulate recollections and colouring-in on specially designed thematic cards (mycolourfulmemories.co.uk/).

The organization Age Exchange, based in Blackheath village in south-east London, supports people living with dementia through person-centred, so-called 'Reminiscence Arts' interventions. The centre offers day-care services for people living with a dementia diagnosis and their carers, as well as weekly reminiscence and arts-based group activities. It has a library and a café in addition to spaces for individual and group activities. Initially piloted with people living in 12 residential care homes with support from Guy's and St Thomas' Charity, a three-year pilot project was carefully monitored and produced a series of reports with six key findings:

1. Wellbeing of participants with dementia increased by 42%, and positive behaviour increased by 25% as a result of taking part in Reminiscence Arts activity.

2. Group Reminiscence Arts sessions significantly improved the quality of life of people living with dementia in the first 50 minutes.

3. Engaging in Reminiscence Arts has the potential to enhance care home residents' lives by improving their connection to both the place they currently live and to spaces of memory and imagination.

4. Attending a Group Reminiscence Arts session steadily and significantly improves the quality of life of people living with dementia week on week over a 24-week period.

5. Reminiscence Arts is a fusion of different art forms and reminiscence practices that is unique to Age Exchange. It responds to the interests, life histories, abilities and needs of participants living with dementia.

6. Group Reminiscence Arts sessions create a social space for all those who participate, including artists, carers and

people living with dementia. By including a range of art forms, Reminiscence Arts creates the opportunity for a wide range of social, cultural and aesthetic interactions.[1]

Similar findings are echoed in various research publications that have explored the value of group interaction through arts interventions (see, for example, Patterson & Perlstein, 2011).

As well as the community-focussed social enterprise initiatives mentioned above, some health authorities are engaged in providing new facilities, such as an in-house 'film booth' in the middle of a ward at Hull Royal Infirmary that simulates the cinema-going experience. It shows footage of Yorkshire throughout the decades to help patients with memory problems. According to the StaffAid nursing agency website:

> *The film booth, complete with cinema seats and a giant screen, has been set up in the middle of Ward 80 to help people reminisce about their past and share memories of growing up in the city. Ward 80 is the Progression to Discharge Unit where patients recovering from recent illness spend time recuperating before they are discharged home with support or to a care home. The cinema helps to keep people mobile, encouraging them to move around the ward to prevent muscle wastage and get back into a more normal routine following a hospital stay.* (https:// www.staffaid.co.uk/?s=hospital+cinema)

---

1 See Final Report of the Evaluation, December 2015 (by Royal Holloway, University of London), Quantitative Evaluation (Royal Holloway University of London – January 2016) C.E.A Report, October 2015 (by Simetrica). Retrieved from https://www.age-exchange.org.uk/what-we-do/inspired-caring/radiql/. Accessed on June 21, 2019.

Regional film archives have been increasingly active in providing resources to assist with memory work in various settings, be it a hospital ward, a nursing home or a day-care centre. Yorkshire Film Archive's award-winning series of DVDs has been developed in consultation with health-care professionals, older people, care workers, volunteer carers and families of people living with a dementia diagnosis. The DVDs contain selected archive footage organized by themes such as holidays, domestic life, schooldays, working life, sport and leisure.[2] The collection is available for purchase from the archive; their latest theme, developed in association with Age UK, focusses on life on the home front in the Second World War and the early post-war period. In a similar vein, following a series of workshops using old films to stimulate memories and autobiographical stories, Screen Archive South East has produced a range of DVDs using archive footage. Some of these focus on individual towns and places, others on themes such as childhood, weddings and the seaside.[3] Inspired by these initiatives, we created two DVDs to accompany our *Cinema, Memory and Wellbeing* toolkit, with the help of North West Film Archive and amateur film collectors on Merseyside and in Greater Manchester. We have used these in a variety of ways in our different projects, including to recreate the filmgoing experience of the 1940s and 1950s, where audiences were accustomed to watching newsreels as part of a programme of films that included a leading 'A' film and a supporting 'B' film. As discussed in more detail in Chapter 1, we even included an interval where ice creams and retro sweets were handed out by care workers dressed as usherettes (see Fig. 1.4, Chapter 1).

---

2 http://www.yorkshirefilmarchive.com/buy-memory-bank. Accessed on July 9, 2019.

3 http://screenarchive.brighton.ac.uk/collection/1473/.

THE POWER OF REMINISCENCE

Reminiscence is the most important psychological task of older people (Touhy & Jett, 2016, p. 68)

Reminiscing – the sharing of life experiences, memories and stories from the past – can have many goals, ranging from the promotion of pleasant memories that improve quality of life to increased socialization, from mental stimulation and improved communication to enhanced personal growth (Touhy & Jett, 2016). Various research projects claim that activities that involve people in talking about their past lives have demonstrable benefits in terms of altered mood if continued over time, with people becoming more positive in their outlook and, in the short term at least, being happier (see, for example, Elias, Neville, & Scott, 2015). Reminiscence therapy has been widely shown to improve depressive symptoms, mood, cognitive functions, social disturbance, self-esteem, feelings of loneliness and life satisfaction (Hus & Wang, 2009). Various studies from a range of professional health disciplines argue that the use of reminiscing not only expands communication and sociability in older adults, but it also contributes to improved elder self-esteem, life satisfaction and overall quality of life (see, for example, Tamura-Lis, 2017). It has proven beneficial for elders and their caregivers in assisted living environments (Assisted Living Today, online), and for nurses, reminiscence therapy can be used in assessment and to foster greater understanding of their patients (Tamura-Lis, 2017). According to Charles N. Lewis (1971):

> *Reminiscence seems to involve first of all the process of memory, with the added action property of reaching out to infuse others with these memories. The recent psychological literature confirms the ability of memory*

> *to color one's past to suit present needs and points out*
> *how influencing others can be motivated by the need to*
> *reduce discrepancies in one's own self-concept, as in*
> *dissonance reduction* (Lewis, 1971, p. 240)

Reminiscence therapy has been used extensively since the 1960s by professional practitioners such as psychologists, nursing staff, social workers and recreational therapists. It has been a popular treatment and intervention for older adults because of its nonpharmacological nature. Reminiscence therapy has been shown to have a positive impact on older patients with and without mental health problems (Elias et al., 2015). Chao et al. (2006) explored reminiscence therapy by using participant observation as their method of study, an approach that we believe provides important 'evidence' in our own projects. The information collected included the personal characteristics of the residents, the content of the reminiscence, settings and triggers or catalysts, the verbal and non-verbal reactions of residents and the thoughts and feelings of researchers. Triggers for reminiscence included *auditory* and *visual* stimuli, a finding that was a central motivation for our own projects, which harness the power of both music and film, giving results that we believe are greater than the sum of their parts.

Music has been shown to stimulate autobiographical memory recall among older people, and in turn reduce anxiety (Foster & Valentine, 1998). In 2018, the cross-disciplinary Commission on Dementia and Music concluded that 'music offers a potential lifeline for people with dementia, their carers and loved ones, one which can sometimes be unmatched by other interventions' (International Longevity Centre-UK, accessed online). Moving images, as Kuhn (2002) has demonstrated, stimulate a wealth of memories about the film in question and the contexts in which it was watched in the past.

By combining music with moving images in the form of reminiscence activities for older people, particularly those in long-term care, but also those living with a dementia diagnosis, we believe these positive benefits can be further consolidated and amplified. In addition to emotional wellbeing benefits (what academics often refer to as 'positive affect'), this can lead to physical improvements, such as stimulation of the immune system, as has been studied in relation to musical interventions (Fancourt, Ockleford, & Belai, 2014).

In 2017, the Cochrane Library produced 'Reminiscence therapy for dementia', a systematic review of the research literature on the subject, building on reviews that it had already produced in 1998 and 2005 (cochranelibrary.com). Commenting on the publication of the review in 2018, health blogger Bob Woods, a dementia care practitioner and researcher, found a step change had occurred in the quality and quantity of research studies available. Woods states:

> *We were able to include 16 well-conducted studies in our analyses, involving a total of 1,749 people with dementia. We anticipated that the effects of reminiscence therapy might be seen on measures of quality of life, interaction and communication and on mood, as well as on cognitive function. Where family carers were involved, we considered the quality of relationship between person with dementia and carer could be influenced, and that carer stress might be reduced.* (evidentlycochrane.net. Accessed online July 2019).

Woods was initially disappointed with the results: according to the studies, there were no consistent benefits or improvements in the quality of life, but for studies using the accepted Mini Mental State Exam (MMSE), 'the benefit was roughly equivalent to preventing 6 months decline in cognitive function in the average person with dementia' (evidentlycochrane.net, July 2019).[4] He concluded that 'there is some evidence that reminiscence therapy can improve quality of life, cognition, communication and possibly mood in people with dementia in some circumstances.' The possible reduction in 'carer stress' referred to in the above quote is worthy of a brief aside. The benefits of reminiscence activities using film and music for boosting carer resilience have been one of the unexpected consequences of our various projects in Brazil and on Merseyside. Powerful testimonies from carers and health professionals who we worked with, discussed in more detail in Chapters 1 and 3, evidenced improvements in their own emotional wellbeing as a result of involvement in the projects, as well as increased job satisfaction and expansion of their skill sets. In recent years there has been an increasing awareness of the importance of 'caring for the carers'. A study conducted by the MHA care home group and Anglia Ruskin and Nottingham Universities into the benefits of music therapy focussed on the 'community wellbeing' of residential homes, which is obviously highly dependent on the individual wellbeing not just of the residents but the staff (Atkinson, Bagnall, Corcoran, South, & Curtis, 2019).[5] This boost to wellbeing for carers can, in turn,

---

4 The MMSE has become one of the standard ways for medical professionals to measure cognitive decline in dementia; in the UK, it has been complemented by the development of Addenbrooke's Cognitive Examination (ACE) which uses a similar range of questions.

5 Atkinson et al. (2019) persuasively advocate an understanding of community wellbeing framed through relationality rather than individual subjectivity. As the authors state, 'if community is taken to be more than the sum of its parts then, as a social grouping, assessment needs to capture aspects of life, including wellbeing, as they are lived and experienced together […]. Assessing wellbeing in terms of this collective aspect of life demands a different approach from assessing individual or aggregated population scale individual subjective wellbeing.'

help reduce staff sickness and improve the productivity and retention of staff, with attendant cost savings. Non-professional carers looking after family members in the home, or volunteer carers, can also implement reminiscence activities, even on a one-to-one basis, thus improving their skill sets, resilience and confidence, and enabling them to look after loved ones for longer and delaying the latter's institutionalization. This has been recognized by the *House of Memories* programme; their app is designed to help carers collect digital sounds and images to stimulate reminiscence and 'grow' the memory bank of the people they are caring for. The Mental Health Foundation provides a 'Carers Checklist', which can be downloaded free of charge, and which facilitates monitoring the wellbeing of both the cared for and the carer, and assessing the effectiveness of interventions on both parties.[6] One of the stated aims of the 'Checklist' is to 'evaluate the impact of service provision on carer burden and carer satisfaction, both for individuals and for groups of service users.' This tool could thus be used in tandem with the toolkit that accompanies this book to evaluate the benefits of the latter's use in the organization of film- and music-related interventions for both carers and the people they care for.

MOVIES, MUSIC AND MEMORY: UNDERPINNING RESEARCH

Memory inhabits, colours, and even forms, our inner worlds. (Kuhn, 1995, p. 159)

Movies and music were the two most popular art forms of the twentieth century, with films and songs, as well as their

---

6 It can be accessed here: https://www.mentalhealth.org.uk/publications/carers-checklist.

performers, often transcending cultural and national differences and boundaries to become transnational, global phe-
nomena. In arts and humanities research, there is a developing
academic literature on the cultural, social and cognitive processes involved in acts of remembering. In our own areas of
research in the fields of film and music, reminiscence has been
of key importance in developing histories of cinema-going and
music and media consumption, drawing on interview material
provided by those who often vividly recall going to the movies
or dance venues or to hear bands, pop groups and musicians
performing. Researchers often start out with a specific purpose;
in our work, for example, to see if people remember a particular star, as in the case of Lisa's work on the Brazilian film star
Carmen Miranda (Shaw, 2013), or if viewers remember a
particular TV series (Hallam, 2005) or whether they can recall
particular music venues, as in the case of Sara's work on Liverpool's musical spaces (Cohen, & Kronenburg, 2018).
Annette Kuhn's work on memories of cinema-going in 1930s'
Britain, *An Everyday Magic: Cinema and Cultural Memory*
(2002), holds a particularly important place in the field because
of the in-depth attention paid to memory and how it is
constituted. Kuhn conducted interviews with older people in
four UK locations to inform her examination of both the cultural and psychical processes involved in the research participants' memories of cinema-going and to create what she terms
an ethnohistory. Seventy-eight people were selected for the
study, around half of whom were interviewed on their own,
the others accompanied by partners, friends and/or residential
care staff. Taken together, the interviews reveal a history of
cinema-going that demonstrates the importance of film in
people's everyday lives, not through memories of particular
movies, but through the recollection of particular details, such
as walking the same route to the cinema many times, certain
kinds of experiences at the movies such as being frightened by

horror films, and going dancing as part of a night out that also featured a movie. We want to use Kuhn's work to open up a discussion about memory and reminiscence and to think about the role of imagination and creativity in the production of memory and its relationship to sustaining a sense of self.

In an earlier study, *Family Secrets: Acts of Memory and Imagination*, Kuhn analyzes her own responses to photographs from her childhood, subjecting her memories to in-depth analysis and considering why the pictures that she is looking at often hold meanings that are rarely immediately apparent. She writes that '[m]emories evoked by a photo do not simply spring out of the image itself, but are generated in a network, an intertext, of discourses that shift between past and present, spectator and image, and between all these cultural contexts, historical moments' (1995, p. 14). Memory is rooted in the personal experiences of individuals, but it is highly coloured by both collective and public memory. Collective memory is constituted by the forms of speech and communication used to share memories amongst a particular generation and group of people such as, in our first project, people from Merseyside who were teenagers in the 1950s. We found that this group of older people share similar forms of speech and expressions to communicate their memories of aspects of urban life, such as working on the docks, travel on the overhead railway locally known as 'the dockers umbrella', factory work, going 'into town' (the city centre) to particular night clubs like the famous Cavern Club, specific kinds of food (like the local stew known as 'scouse') and drink, and other locally and time-specific attitudes and ideas about topics such as sport and fashion. Overlying but also constituting these collective memories is what is frequently termed public or official memory, a memory often sustained by national myths, such as the political message that those growing up in the 1950s 'had never had it so good', even though the inner cities of the UK, Liverpool amongst them, had areas of extreme deprivation and poverty. National myths are often embalmed in cinema newsreels about historical events such as the coronation of Elizabeth II in 1953, and increasingly in television programmes made about past times, all of which inflect personal memory in various ways. For Kuhn, memory is a personal activity, a process that is 'staged through words, both spoken and written, in images of many kinds and also in sounds' (1995, p. 157). As we noted at the beginning of this section, Kuhn argues that: 'Memory inhabits, colours, and even forms, our inner worlds' (1995, p. 159). When we are working with people's memories, by stimulating them to remember past times, places and emotions, we are helping them to keep alive their inner worlds. It is this rationale that has underpinned all our projects.

Kuhn's work highlights the value of using visual material to access various aspects of memory among her ageing research participants, yet, in spite of the popularity of cinema-going and movie watching for much of the twentieth century, there is scant evidence that the research underpinning these therapeutic benefits of communal film viewing is being drawn on or developed in the context of health-care settings such as day-care centres and nursing homes. Our own projects have therefore sought inspiration in Kuhn's pioneering work and have consciously set out to develop its practical aspects and applications. In contrast, when we consider music in third-age care, there are multiple ways in which it is being used: music therapy, music-making and music as entertainment, amongst others. Music-making activities are widely used for therapeutic purposes, being employed to combat depression (Costa, Ockelford, & Hargreaves, 2018); as a form of sedation (Johnson & Taylor, 2011); and as a trigger for reminiscence (Istvandity, 2017). The prominence given to the documentary film *Alive Inside* (Rossato-Bennett, 2014), discussed in more detail below, is a reflection of the increased media coverage and cultural engagement around music's therapeutic potential, especially in later life. This, in turn, has prompted the growth of initiatives with therapeutic aims, such as *Music and Memory* and *Playlist for Life*, also explored below, as well as solidifying the notion of musical activities such as singalongs and performances as synonymous with a happy, healthy caring environment.

The past few decades have seen an increase in collective music-making and listening activities within dementia care. This has become particularly prominent through the publicity given to charities such as *Music and Memory* (https://musicandmemory.org) and *Playlist for Life* (https://www.playlistforlife.org.uk), and thanks to films such as the award-winning documentary *Alive Inside*. This film recounts the experiences of *Music and Memory*'s founder, social worker Dan Cohen, as he seeks to demonstrate music's ability to combat memory loss and restore a sense of self to those suffering cognitive impairment against the background of a US health-care system that is failing many of its older citizens. In the film, neurologist Oliver Sacks states: 'I have seen deeply demented patients weep or shiver as they listen to music [...] Once one has seen such as response, one knows that there is still a self to be called upon, even if the music and only the music, can do the calling.' Music's ability to connect listeners with their past selves is particularly important for those living with dementia. The power of music to connect with listeners in such an impactful way has positive ramifications not only for the listener but also for carers and family members, who are able to glimpse a self that is so fractured from the present that it is sometimes feared lost forever.

A common thread in the academic literature about music and memory is music's ability to connect not only to recollections of the past but also to a person's sense of identity and personal life stories that are linked to those musical moments. In her summarized account of the research on music and reminiscence, Lauren Istvandity concludes that: 'Studies across the domains of psychology and sociology demonstrate that music can effectively trigger autobiographical memories with strong emotional content and that an individual's personal memories of music are closely tied to their self-identity and life story' (Istvandity, 2017, p. 19). This reminiscence allows not only access to personal memories but also to the relationships and social connections that those memories evoke; Terrence Hays and Victor Minichiello observed this in their 2005 study, noting how music connected their participants 'to others who may no longer be living, and may also validate memories, give meaning to life, and bring a greater sense of spirituality' (Hays & Minichiello, 2005, p. 449). The power of music in triggering memory is deeply personal and autobiographical in nature; particular songs may be meaningful to more than one person, but the emotion and memories entwined with the songs may vary greatly.

Music is a catalyst for remembering particular events, people, emotions and places. Key factors appear to be the autobiographical salience of the music for the individual and how 'nostalgia-prone' the individual is found to be (Barrett et al., 2010; Gallotti & Frith, 2013). Researchers interested in music and memory have identified a so-called 'reminiscence bump' or 'memory bump', whereby music from an older person's youth and adolescence is recognized more often, with more facts known about it, and evokes more specific autobiographical memories and strong emotions than music from later in life. According to Rathbone, Moulin, and Conway (2008), between the ages of 12 and 22 years, and coinciding with the 'reminiscence bump', a stable and enduring sense of self emerges.[7] The storage of autobiographical memory is not consistent through time, rather it increases through seasons of change such as adolescence, as the memories from this period are more easily accessible (Platz, Kopiez, Hasselhorn, & Wolf, 2015, p. 238). Based on this research that sheds light on which areas of memory are more accessible via musical stimulus, and taking inspiration from the *Playlist for Life* project, which researches the music that an individual would have listened to in the past and seeks to create a very personal playlist for them to access, we have been increasingly focussed in our choices of soundtracks for our various projects. In our project in partnership with the day-care centre in the Speke district of Liverpool, run by Company Matters4U, for example, we tried to recreate a feeling of the 1950s' cinema-going experience. Our colleague from the Department of Music, Sara Cohen, assembled playlists of popular music from that decade to accompany the arrival of our guests and to provide interest during the interval between the two halves of the film screening event (see Chapter 1).

As well as being a catalyst, music is also considered to be a reservoir for memory; it is not just a trigger creating an emotional flashback, but a means for actually storing the emotions connected to and associated with a piece of music (van Djick, 2006, p. 359). Music thus functions like a deep well from which we can draw upon our past as it is entangled with our sense of self and our emotions; it is a resource that enables listeners to mentally time travel to a specific place or experience from the past. There is a connective-ness to not only the actual memory of the music or song but also the context in which it was experienced, and the emotions

---

7 Notions of self and social identity connected with music have also been explored by Bennett (2013); Frith (1996); MacDonald, Miell, and Wilson (2005).

associated with that moment. These contexts can include public and private moments, as well as allowing people to situate themselves in these past moments, locating the self within the broader cultural affiliations of collective memory that we discussed above. In our Liverpool projects, for example, many of the care home residents and day centre participants remembered the songs performed by Carmen Miranda in her films, as well as talking about their personal emotions associated with particular songs, as we discuss in more detail in Chapter 1. This was equally the case in our projects in Petrópolis, Brazil, even amongst people with mild dementia-related cognitive impairment, as discussed in Chapter 3. Kindell, Burrow, Wilkinson, and David Keady (2014) highlight the importance of these personal records of experiences and the act of recounting them; they argue that this is particularly important for helping older people to articulate a biographical connection between past and pre-sent lives, and that these connections, in part, enable the preservation of the person's identity and affirm a sense of agency and the self. This becomes increasingly important when we consider those living with a dementia diagnosis as it is the link between past and present lives that becomes frayed, and this biographical remembering, even in small ways, can be significant in helping to hold these intangible threads of the self in place.

The role of music in the stimulation or preservation of memory extends beyond the act of hearing. Musical objects can also act as stimuli for memory, much like NML's 'memory boxes', discussed above (Bennett & Rogers, 2016; Cohen, 2014, 2016; Pickering & Keightley, 2015). Researchers have shown how record sleeves, concert tickets, posters and other forms of musical memorabilia are impor-tant in prompting conversations about past memories and allow for the development of connections between people via objects that connect to specific musical experiences. Development of music streaming services such as Spotify, and the accessibility of music on digital media such as YouTube, often means that the importance of physical, music-related objects is neglected. However, these objects can act as a gateway to musical memory and offer insights into important and significant stories of the self. Music and musical artefacts have a particular significance in work with older age groups because of their ability to generate shared, collective memories from the past by connecting our present selves to past selves and supporting narratives of our personal identities in the present. This connective-ness is highly important in supporting relationships between people in a given context, such as a nursing home, and between older people and the wider society around them, including their younger relatives.

Beyond using music listening and music-related artefacts as a resource for stimulating memory, music-making is also widely shown to create or enhance connective-ness. Gallotti and Frith refer to the concept of 'we-ness' – the 'we-ness' of singing and making music, as well as of listening to and experiencing music, as a group. They state: 'This first-person plural perspective captures the viewpoint of individuals engaged in social interactions and thus expands each individual's potential for social understanding and action' (2013, p. 160). We have all at some level experienced this 'we-ness' through music, be that the experience of feeling the bass pump through our bodies at a music gig, or the unity of singing together in a choir or in a crowd at a football match. This 'we-ness' supports the individual person's potential for relating to others and for being active in their connections to other people; this bond and the community building that is enabled through creating music together is discussed in more detail in Chapter 2.

The effectiveness of shared singing as a tool for increasing wellbeing amongst those with a cognitive impairment, as well as for raising morale amongst carers who take part in the singing, has been demonstrated in qualitative studies (see, for example, Osman, Tischler, & Schneider, 2016). The evident entertainment value and pleasure generated by group musical activities has led to numerous initiatives, such as *Singing for the Brain*, a service provided by the Alzheimer's Society that uses singing and other activities to bring together people with dementia or memory loss, and *A Choir in Every Care Home*, funded and initiated by the Baring Foundation. In its care of those living with dementia, the MHA care home group is leading the way in the use of music therapy – described by the British Association for Music Therapy as 'an established psychological clinical intervention, which is delivered by [...] registered music therapists to help people whose lives have been affected by injury, illness or disability through support-ing their psychological, emotional, cognitive, physical, communicative and social needs' (online). A study of the benefits of music therapy involving the MHA group and Anglia Ruskin and Nottingham Universities showed quite dramatically that it had a beneficial effect on the symptoms of dementia both during the therapy and beyond.[8] Singing can be stimulated in any group setting, be it a day centre or a care home, with very little effort or cost involved. Company Matters4U, a group of day-care centres that we worked with in Liverpool, achieve this by running regular karaoke sessions that prove extremely popular with their service users. Some classical music institutions, such as the Hallé Orchestra in Manchester, discussed in more detail in Chapter 2, run pro-jects that seek to create new music together with those living

---

8 https://www.artshealthandwellbeing.org.uk/case-studies/music-therapy-and-dementia.

in local care facilities.[9] Music establishes and maintains interpersonal relationships and a sense of self not solely as a tool for reminiscence but as a lived experience in the present. Music is the most social of all art forms, and this makes it particularly effective for use with older people as they are at a much higher risk of social isolation than other age groups. Music is a way of encouraging social interaction, by making music or singing together, or sharing listening experiences and related memories. In Chapter 2 we will demonstrate how our work explores the importance of this social aspect of music-making and will highlight music's role in supporting healthy ageing.

REMINISCENCE, NOSTALGIA AND DEMENTIA

Reminiscence is a very effective tool for connecting with people living with a dementia diagnosis, since they are more likely to recall things from a distant past than recent times. Reminiscence thus allows them to make use of a skill they still have, rather than dwelling on what they have lost, fostering a sense of confidence, self-esteem and competence. The fact that they can actively share something with others, instead of depending on them passively, and actually inform and interest others, gives them a sense of dignity and purpose. For those living with dementia, evidence shows that musical memory is preserved and that it can be reliably and quantitatively assessed via the observation of behaviour (Cuddy & Duffin, 2005). Even for people with advanced Alzheimer's disease, the musical memory areas of the brain remain intact and functioning (Jacobsen et al., 2015). Reminiscence projects

9 https://www.halle.co.uk/education/community-projects/work-with-older-people/. Accessed on September 29, 2019.

that use music as a trigger thus chime with the government's national strategy 'Living Well with Dementia'. Group reminiscence has the added potential of fostering connections between people from different backgrounds (social classes, religions, sexualities, races, nationalities etc.); beneficially, it can often also give rise to previously unknown commonalities, and allow carers – particularly professionals but sometimes even family members – to find out new things about people's pasts, their likes and dislikes, to think about them in a different light and to identify topics that can be explored in greater depth in future interactions. A carer may do a little research on the Internet about a film, film star or singers that someone remembers, or try to find images of a local cinema that he or she used to frequent. Reminiscence in the home context or involving family members of someone living in residential care is a powerful tool for bringing families together. Shared experiences like this foster a sense of collective wellbeing, strengthening connections and a sense of community/family and belonging.

One of the issues that reminiscence therapy raises that is rarely discussed in the academic literature is that, as well as recalling good times from the past, distressing memories of unhappy life events and difficult times can be evoked. Nostalgia is an emotional process that can accompany autobiographical memories and gives rise primarily – but not exclusively – to positive 'affect' (a term that academics often use to refer to emotions), being able to counteract negative feelings, such as sadness and loneliness. Barrett et al. (2010) argue that music-evoked nostalgia can trigger both positive and negative emotional experiences, and that nostalgia can be bittersweet at times, involving a 'blend of positive (e.g. joy) and negative (e.g. sadness) emotions' (Barrett et al., 2010, p. 400). Many people in caring roles who took part in our projects expressed concern about bringing back painful memories and sparking negative emotions in people who are naturally vulnerable due to their age and/or diagnosis. It is important to remember, however, that emotional reactions – including tears – are not necessarily a bad thing, provided that they are responded to with sensitivity. On one occasion in Brazil, in the course of the project at the Fazenda Inglesa GP practice, a lady in her 80s with early-stage dementia began to cry when she saw a film clip of the star Carmen Miranda singing 'Mamãe, eu quero' ('Mummy, I want some'). She said it was the song her mother sang to her and her siblings to get them to sleep when she was a little girl. Lisa was initially very concerned about her visible reaction, and immediately spoke to the lady's carer and consent-giver (her daughter), suggesting they both took a break from the session. Both mother and daughter were keen to continue, however, making it clear that although the song had moved her deeply and reduced her to tears, the older lady's memories were happy ones and the experience had been entirely positive. In contrast, in one of our sessions in Liverpool, a participant recalled a house she had lived in where a close relative was murdered. On the advice of her carer, we moved on to discuss the benefits of the new, modern house that she moved to, which fortunately prompted positive memories. In this instance, there seemed little evidence of ongoing distress, but it did raise a question for us about which the research literature says very little. Most studies claim that reminiscence has overwhelmingly positive wellbeing benefits, emphasizing the enhanced coping strategies enabled by reminiscence therapy that allow participants to overcome psychological distress (see, for example, Satorres, Viguer, Fortuna, & Meléndez, 2017).

The Social Care Institute for Excellence's document *Reminiscence for People with Dementia* gives expert guidance on how to communicate well with those living with the disease.[10] It points out, for example, that they might not respond well to direct questions (e.g. Do you remember when…?), and recommends as an alternative that you should begin by sharing a memory yourself, giving clues about what sort of things to talk about, and help the person relax, reassuring them that they need not worry about forgetting or confusing something. The Institute offers a 'Dementia Awareness' e-learning course, described on its website as seeking 'to improve the wellbeing and experience of people with dementia and of the care staff working with them', and as helping carers 'feel more confident in managing challenging situations'. NML's *House of Memories* programme also offers free dementia awareness training, workshops and materials. Its mission statement is a powerful reminder of the benefits of reminiscence for people with the condition and how such activities can help their carers to connect with them:

> *As a museum, we understand that a person's history and memory are of great value and significance – especially for people living with dementia. House of Memories has been developed to support carers in the sharing of memories with people living with dementia, improving communication and focussing on the person rather than the condition (online).*

Before beginning our pilot projects, Lisa attended a *House of Memories* Dementia Awareness Day at the Museum of Liverpool. The trainer stressed that informal dementia carers (such as family members) – who currently number over

---

10 Retrieved from https://www.scie.org.uk/dementia/living-with-dementia/ keeping-active/reminiscence.asp.

850,000 in the UK – are also 'living with dementia'. One-third of us will care for someone with dementia in our lifetime. The trainer underlined the importance of reminiscence sessions in providing pleasurable moments for people with dementia and their family members, and in enabling carers to remember, or discover for the first time, what makes the person they care for 'tick'. He called reminiscence activities 'pathways to interaction', a phrase which has stuck in our minds as we elaborated our various projects, as has the idea of such activities enabling 'moments of connection', which we believe is the key to fostering a sense of wellbeing in people living with dementia in particular.

We hope that the toolkit that we have developed for working with people living with cognitive disorders and/or a dementia diagnosis, both carers and those they care for, will be a useful guide for those unaccustomed to running group activities and will create many 'pathways to interaction'. We also hope that the minimal requirements in terms of resources for running these sessions will inspire people, whether they are a researcher, a professional carer, an individual caring for a relative, a volunteer, a service provider or a policy maker, to have some fun and have a go themselves. In the rest of this book, we discuss the various projects we have undertaken over recent years and the ways we made the contacts that made them possible, beginning in Chapter 1 with our first projects at a residential care home in Liverpool, Merseyside, UK and at the Fazenda Inglesa primary healthcare centre in the city of Petrópolis, Rio de Janeiro State, Brazil.

1

CINEMA, MEMORY AND WELLBEING: PILOT PROJECTS IN LIVERPOOL AND BRAZIL

Lisa Shaw and Julia Hallam

INTRODUCTION

Colleagues at the University of Liverpool, but above all great friends who both had older parents and a passionate commitment to developing projects to engage with and support the local community, in late 2014 Lisa Shaw (Professor of Brazilian Studies) and Julia Hallam (Professor of Film and Media Studies) came up with the idea of combining their interests and teaming up with care homes in the Merseyside area to create the project *Cinema, Memory and Wellbeing*. In this chapter, we explore how our different research interests and approaches have coalesced to inform the development of various linked pilot projects and the toolkit that we have developed for use by care workers and volunteers working in day-care and residential settings. These linked projects use film and music to improve the wellbeing of older people in the UK and Brazil, including those living with a dementia-related cognitive impairment, in nursing home and health-care settings and as part of activities organized for those living independently.

Julia has published books and articles on various aspects of film and media and led research on the relationship between film, place and memory as part of the government-funded Arts and Humanities Research Council 'City in Film' project.[1] While working with amateur filmmaking organizations from Merseyside, Julia was struck by how frequently the filmmakers were asked to show their films to local groups and organizations catering primarily for older people, where they provided a common point of recognition for discussion, reminiscence and social engagement. Wirral-based filmmaker and collector Angus Tilston regularly screened his amateur movies of the city in past times to local groups and in care homes. As Julia says: 'When I discussed the screening of these films with him, he talked about how the films stimulated a collective memory that was often shared by the group and gave them something to talk about. He was convinced that these screenings had a therapeutic benefit'.

Lisa, on the other hand, has published books on Brazilian popular music and cinema, particularly the musical comedy tradition known as *chanchada*, a genre that launched the career of Carmen Miranda in Brazil before she was catapulted to international stardom in Hollywood in the 1940s. During research for her book *Carmen Miranda* (Shaw, 2013), Lisa was struck by the numbers of older fans of the star from all over the world (including her own mother and auntie from Runcorn in North West England!), who were keen to tell her about the therapeutic value of watching one of her films on DVD today. Lisa discovered that all the older

---

1 The project explores the relationship between film, memory and the urban landscape. https://www.liverpool.ac.uk/architecture/research/cava/cityfilm/

fans she interviewed still use Miranda's films and music as a way of enhancing their emotional wellbeing. Their testimonies reveal the ability of musical film to stimulate positive emotions, particularly among older people. One fan in Brazil commented: 'For me, Carmen Miranda's most important legacy was that she always brought joy to people – even today and without being physically present.' Another older Australian fan said: 'Her legacy to the world is in one word – happiness. It is impossible to feel down when you watch her on film.' As British super-fan Ivan Jack succinctly put it in an interview with Lisa: 'She left us all happy. I'll never forget her.' Another fan in Brazil confessed that he particularly listens to her songs or watches her films when he is feeling tired, stressed, angry or sad, adding: 'Carmen has the power to make me quickly feel joyful again, to find peace of mind.'

In her research into the Brazilian musical comedy tradition known as the *chanchada*, Lisa had studied local audiences' identificatory responses to its film stars in the 1940s and 1950s. She had concluded that the success of these films hinged in large part on their ability to engage spectators in identifying with the characters on screen, and the stars who played them, as they constructed their own cultural meanings and sense of selfhood. Drawing on work such as that of Annette Kuhn and Jackie Stacey, she also explored the role of audience memory in cultural constructions of identity, conducting a small parallel study of how older audiences in Brazil today remember their relationship with the home-grown screen idols of their youth. She was particularly inspired by the way that Stacey emphasized in her work the importance of social identities and cultural differences, such as gender, race and class, in determining how audiences of the past and present interpret films and their stars. As Stacey concluded:

> *Stars were as important for cinema spectators as the*
> *narratives of the films in which they appeared. They*
> *offered one of the key sources of pleasure to the*
> *cinema audiences. Stars were the most common*
> *reason given for the choice of film made in the 1940s*
> *by cinema-goers in my research* (Stacey, 1994,
> p. 106)

In her research into film stardom in Brazil, Lisa had explored how the *chanchada* musical comedies sought to attract a wide audience by adopting formulaic elements that appealed to both genders, and to people of different racial and regional backgrounds. She furthermore discovered that in spite of the low-brow connotations of this cinematic tradition, audience members were drawn from a variety of social classes. These films, which are now increasingly available on DVD, thus provided a rich source of material to engage with a vast spectrum of 'third-age' Brazilians today, and particularly those born in the 1930s and 1940s. Those born in later decades were also likely to have seen these films either at the cinema as children, or in their adolescence and early adulthood, when they began to appear on free-to-air television. Carmen Miranda's Hollywood musicals, which Lisa had studied in depth for a book about the star, were also screened in Brazil in the 1940s and 1950s and had huge repercussions in the press.

These research findings gave Lisa the idea of putting her extensive collection of Carmen Miranda films and Brazilian *chanchadas* to good use. Having visited several nursing homes in Merseyside and Cheshire, not least when her father required residential care, Lisa was struck by how television and DVD collections were being under-utilized to stimulate residents cognitively and emotionally. There was clearly a need for a much more interactive experience of film viewing and a creative, dynamic engagement with audio-visual material that could improve the participants' sense of wellbeing. The *Cinema, Memory and Wellbeing* project that we created for use on Merseyside uses a combination of archive film footage of Liverpool and clips from Carmen Miranda's spectacular Hollywood musicals, to trigger memories and spark reminiscences among older, care home audiences. We were keen to explore the emotional wellbeing benefits of group reminiscence of this kind. With the financial support of a University of Liverpool Knowledge Exchange Voucher, in March 2015 we held two pilot *Cinema, Memory and Wellbeing* events for residents of a nursing home in Liverpool. The audience responded enthusiastically to a series of short clips of documentary footage of scenes of the city in the 1950s and early 1960s, as well as excerpts from feature films shot on location in Liverpool. Clearly fascinated by these locations associated with their younger lives, they began to reminisce with each other. Lisa then took the project to Brazil, where she worked with a GP in a practice in the city of Petrópolis, in the state of Rio de Janeiro. With some minor modifications, the methodology proved to be equally effective in eliciting shared reminiscences and wellbeing benefits among older Brazilians. The results of all these projects are discussed in more detail below.

PILOT PROJECT AT A NURSING HOME IN LIVERPOOL

We are always looking for ways to help our residents maintain community connections and feel part of the wider city around them – which this project did.

Representative of the Nursing Home[2]

In England, the care home sector is run primarily by private companies, charities and sometimes the local council who admit older people who are struggling to live independently even with the help of daily carers, relatives and friends. As well as accommodation and meals, these homes provide help with personal and/or nursing care. Admission is usually at the request of the individual in consultation with family members following a needs assessment by a social worker or care manager. We worked with the activities coordinator at a privately owned nursing home in Liverpool to devise a film-related activity tailored to the backgrounds and interests of the residents of the home. Most of them were born and raised in Liverpool during the 1930s; by the 1950s, they were living their young adult lives in a city recovering from the traumas of the Second World War. None of the residents knew each other before coming to the home. Some were born in the docklands, an area alongside the river Mersey and adjacent to the city centre that had been heavily bombed during the war, others in the surrounding inner-city housing estates and nineteenth-century terraces. We were aware that the sense of loss of family members and friends, and the traumas of re-housing in the new satellite estates outside the city, might be triggered during the reminiscence sessions. We were therefore careful in our selection of material, choosing short clips (between 3 and 10 minutes in length) of well-known streets, buildings and beaches from popular British Ealing Studios comedy films such as *The Magnet* (Frend, 1950) and 'social problem' films such as *Violent Playground* (Dearden, 1958), the latter clips focussed, for the most part, on a car chase

---

2 We have chosen to anonymize the nursing home as it has since changed ownership and name three times.

through streets left virtually intact after the air raids. A large number of clips were drawn from amateur footage that focussed on activities such as car racing at Aintree (now known for the Grand National horse race), football (matches at Everton and Liverpool Football Clubs), city centre night clubs, shopping areas and work activities on the docks and in the new factories. Lisa selected spectacular musical numbers from some of Carmen Miranda's most popular Hollywood films that had been screened in Liverpool in the 1940s and subsequently screened on the BBC in the 1970s, such as *Down Argentine Way* (Cummings, 1940), *That Night in Rio* (Cummings, 1941) and *The Gangs All Here* (Berkeley, 1943).

While we were waiting for the necessary Criminal Records Bureau (CRB) checks to be conducted and for approval from the University of Liverpool's Research Ethics Committee, an easily transportable projector and sound system had to be bought that would meet the requirements of screenings planned for Liverpool and Petrópolis. (For the Liverpool screenings, we borrowed a projector screen, but for the Brazilian screenings, Lisa thought she would have to improvise with a large white sheet and hopes of a helping hand or two to hang it on the wall! In the end she managed to borrow a large portable screen.) One of the most challenging aspects of audio-visually stimulated memory work, as the discussions of similar projects in the Introduction reveal, is demonstrating the ways in which it can enhance cognitive engagement and a sense of wellbeing. We therefore decided to record on video the sessions to enable us to reflect on the events, as well as providing us with a permanent, qualitative record of interaction with the participants. We also consulted a Professor of Psychology and Public Mental Health experienced in measuring wellbeing, Professor Rhiannon Corcoran from the Institute of Life and Human Sciences at the

University of Liverpool, who helped us to develop a set of tailored instruments for measuring wellbeing using nationally recognized assessments of cognitive abilities and quality-of-life indicators.[3] With Rhiannon's help, we devised a series of simple questionnaires that required responses from the residents the day before the screening, immediately following the screening and 24 hours later (see Appendix). Our intention, following the conventional way of administering the tests, was to ask the staff at the care home to undertake the first stage with the residents the day before the screening, then to work with care home staff to administer the second questionnaire immediately after the event, and to follow up with the final one on the day after the screening.

Due to the research dimension of the project, we needed to ensure that everyone attending the screening was made aware of, and consented to, being recorded on video, that they knew that individual conversations might be recorded and that we would be asking people to complete questionnaires. We also asked the residents for permission to use their comments and images in any publications that might result from the project, be that in on-line postings or any other form of research dissemination. The activities coordinator kindly undertook the task of helping us to explain the project to everyone and obtaining informed consent. With help from the care assistants, we were then able to administer the wellbeing questionnaires the day before the screening, immediately after each session and the following day, to most of the participants, some of whom had mild cognitive impairments linked to a dementia diagnosis.

Screening films in unknown settings and engaging the audience in discussion about them is part of what teachers of

---

3 https://www.liverpool.ac.uk/institute-of-life-and-human-sciences/staff/ rhiannon-corcoran/. Accessed on October 20, 2019.

film and media arts do; nonetheless, nursing home and day-care settings present particular challenges and opportunities. The practical aspects of preparing to screen the films were discussed with the activities coordinator at the nursing home in Liverpool; we needed to ensure that residents could view the screen comfortably and hear the soundtracks as well as interact with us and each other. The large residents lounge was made available, which ensured that all those wanting to participate could be seated comfortably. Power points, extension cables and other trailing wires had to be secured to prevent any tripping hazards or accidents. The projector and the presenter had to be carefully positioned to avoid obstructing vision and maximize the size of the image. We then offered a film and media student keen to gain some experience for his CV the opportunity to video the proceedings; we also had a handheld sound recorder to capture discussions with individuals.

CAPTURING WELLBEING BENEFITS IN A NURSING HOME SETTING

We decided that we would aim to recreate the cinema-going experience of the 1950s a little more closely by emulating a 'newsreel-plus-feature-film' format, albeit only using short clips of films of between 3 and 10 minutes in length to help keep the audience's attention and allow for immediate inter-action after the clips. The first session at the nursing home ran relatively smoothly. The audience responded enthusiastically to the short documentary scenes of the city as well as excerpts from feature films shot on location in Liverpool. Clearly fascinated by these locations associated with their younger lives, the residents began to reminisce with each other, with the care staff and the two of us. Their reminiscences covered a

wide range of topics, with frequent references to the neighbourhoods they had grown up in and their leisure activities,
including going to the cinema, dancing and visits to the city
centre, as well as various jobs they had undertaken during
their younger lives. After an interval for tea and biscuits, the
Liverpool scenes were followed by the Carmen Miranda clips;
many of the residents remembered the songs she performed on
screen, with some even joining in and singing along. After a
chat about Carmen's impact on women's fashions in the
1940s and 1950s, care workers helped us to administer the
second wellbeing questionnaire. The staff from the home also
administered the third and final questionnaire the following
day. (A copy of the questionnaire can be found in the
Appendix.) Two weeks later, the *Cinema, Memory and
Wellbeing* session was repeated with another group at the
home.

The two sessions created a wealth of information which
was analyzed to inform the development of the project and the
accompanying 'best-practice' toolkit, designed to enable
activities coordinators, carers and health professionals to
optimize the benefits of using films to stimulate memories and
reminiscence and an attendant improved sense of wellbeing,
among older people. By filming the audience's reactions and
interactions on video, we gathered valuable evidence of the
wellbeing benefits of the film events, such as participants
becoming increasingly animated, smiling and laughing, chatting animatedly with each other, and one initially very shy
lady even breaking into an almost word-perfect rendition of a
Carmen Miranda song! These impressions were backed up by
the feedback obtained from the wellbeing questionnaires, fil-
led in by all 16 participants with help from ourselves and the
care assistants. The questionnaires sought to measure four
aspects of wellbeing: current satisfaction with life; self-esteem
(Q2, 'my life has been worthwhile'); happiness at the moment

of response; and anxiety levels. Participants were asked to indicate their response on a scale graduated from 1 to 100%, where 1 = totally disagree and 100 = totally agree. In addition, we wanted to gauge their response to the film clips: did the scenes featuring recognizable places prompt memories about past times? did they stimulate happy memories or less happy times? did the Carmen Miranda films prompt happy memories or memories of less happy times? (see Appendix for full details of this particular questionnaire format). Of the 16 participants, we were only able to collect responses from the day before, the day of the screening and the following day from eight of them, although we did have responses for two of the three days from another five respondents. Analyzing these results proved to be difficult, not least how to interpret the responses to the sliding scales on the questionnaire itself. Residents found it too difficult to complete the questionnaires alone; those of us that were helping them to complete it often had to guess at a point on the sliding scales that seemed indicative of their responses. Nonetheless, there was some indication that after the screening, residents felt a little less anxious and the following day, as well as reduced anxiety levels for some participants, for a few people there seemed to be a notable increase in their self-esteem.

While these results are in many ways questionable as evidence of changes in overall wellbeing, the additional questions eliciting responses to the film clips themselves also indicated that people enjoyed the screenings and, that whilst not always stimulating happy memories, the clips often brought to the fore aspects of their lives that they had forgotten. The questionnaire responses did, however, support our video recordings and recorded conversations with people, confirming that while we had not got everything 'right' in terms of our choices of material (particularly in the case of historical footage of Liverpool, where images of war-time damage and housing renewal were still in evidence in the background of some of footage), for the most part residents had found that the screenings brought back memories of happy times and were enjoyable and relaxing. Based on these results, Lisa developed a programme of edited clips to show at the Fazenda Inglesa primary care health centre in the city of Petrópolis, Rio de Janeiro state, Brazil, discussed in more detail in Chapter 3.

Some six months after the two sessions at the nursing home in Liverpool, we returned there at the request of the activities coordinator to repeat the event. Some of those who had initially participated wanted to attend again, so we incorporated new film clips. In addition, we added some related activities; since during the earlier sessions held there many participants had reminisced about their cinema-going experiences in their younger lives, Julia created a folder of photocopied photographs of Liverpool's cinemas in the 1950s and passed these around the audience, asking them to help us identify them and talk about where exactly they were located. Many of the residents found images of their local cinema and talked vividly about the films they had seen there, their favourite stars (both British and Hollywood), as well as other experiences associated with that period of their lives. We also took along some simple costumes and props that recalled those used by Carmen Miranda in the clips we screened – the ladies were keen to try on two elaborately decorated turbans we had commissioned from a local maker of carnival costumes and have their photographs taken, and a couple of gentlemen enthusiastically played the maracas during the musical numbers. We found this ludic dimension to be particularly useful in stimulating laughter and encouraging people to talk. On this occasion we opted not to include any wellbeing questionnaires, given the difficulties we had encountered with delivering and interpreting them, but instead filmed the event and the interactions it led to, on video. Once again, this qualitative data clearly evidenced, in our view, the power of film used in this short-clip, interactive format, to elicit group reminiscence, animated conversation, lively interaction and plenty of laughter. We feel strongly that such results speak for themselves, and that the use of questionnaires would have detracted from the enjoyment of this event, feelings that were to be proved right when Lisa tried to administer questionnaires at the 'Memory Film Club', as we discuss in Chapter 3. Instead, we focussed on getting the carers' views, and at the end of this project with the nursing home we interviewed the staff about their impressions of the project. They gave very positive responses, not only in terms of the benefits it had brought to residents, but because they thought their input had been valued by the residents, fostering trust and friendship between the colleagues and between them and those they care for. A representative of the home said:

> *It was great to introduce our resident group to new and interesting people and encourage conversation, interest and social engagement... The project was also of genuine interest to the staff supporting our residents and encouraged reminiscence across generations.*

FLYING DOWN TO RIO: TAKING THE PROJECT TO BRAZIL

As we mentioned in the Introduction, of Brazil's total population of 205 million, over 7 million are aged over 65 years, and a rapid decline in fertility since the 1960s and increased life expectancy has contributed to an ageing population (https://www.indexmundi.com/brazil/). The Family Health

Programme (PSF – *Programa Saúde da Família*) is a national
public health programme, introduced in Brazil 1991 as part of
a reform of the health care sector, aimed at promoting health
and disease prevention for everyone and implementing a
national policy for primary care. It places emphasis on the
health of families as a whole, rather than individuals, and is
organized around multidisciplinary Family Health Teams,
formed by a core of professionals such as physicians, nurses,
dentists, psychologists and social workers, as well as so-called
community health agents (ACS – *agentes comunitários de
saúde*). The PACS programme for training and deploying
ACSs was also introduced in 1991, whereby individuals who
live in a given community are employed to encourage local
people to make use of the health facilities (each being
responsible for around 120 families). The ACSs are lay health
workers, said to be inspired by the barefoot doctors programme in China. They are not certified to practice medicine
or nursing but have the primary task of gathering information
on the health status of their small community by means of a
close relationship with it. Agents should live in the community
and are supervised by a doctor or nurse. They carry out home
visits, building good relationships with the local population
and gathering information that can help the health clinic
assess the main health challenges in the community.

Having spoken to friends who work as ACSs in the city of
Petrópolis, Rio de Janeiro state, Lisa became increasingly
aware of the lack of tools and training that they have at their
disposal, particularly as regards engagement with older people
in the community. They tend to feel overburdened, undervalued and inadequately resourced. Lisa presented the project
to the GP responsible for the clinic where her ACS friends
work, the Fazenda Inglesa primary care practice, who
acknowledged that the idea of social prescribing (discussed in
the Introduction) is gaining currency in Brazil at an academic

level, but as yet has not trickled down to praxis. He was keen to explore with his team of six ACSs and a practice nurse the possibility of developing arts-based wellbeing activities for his older patients. Working with the GP and a team of six ACSs at the Fazenda Inglesa practice, Lisa adapted the project piloted on Merseyside, drawing on her large collection of Brazilian musical comedy films.

As a specialist in Brazilian popular cinema from the 1940s and 1950s, Lisa developed an audio-visual presentation composed of clips from musical comedy films from that era, including a mixture of musical/dance sequences, scenes shot on location and comic dialogue sequences featuring famous stars from the 1950s. She included male and female stars from different racial and regional backgrounds to maximize the chances of audience identification, and included both low-brow and high-brow locations in the city of Rio de Janeiro, where the films were set and shot. Screenings were held for 68 over-65s, in groups of 20 or so, who were users of the Fazenda Inglesa practice. The local church kindly let the sessions be held in its hall, adjacent to the health practice, and Lisa took the portable projection and recording equipment from the UK, just needing to borrow a large portable screen from the GP himself (see Fig. 1.1). These were interactive events, and following each clip, lasting no more than five minutes, Lisa posed open questions to the audience, to stimulate responses and interaction between them, also prompted by the ACSs, who were dotted around the audience. The GP was keen to actively participate, offering to record the audience's verbal interactions and comments on video, as well as recording other physical reactions, such as smiling and laughter, singing and movement to the music. This capturing of physical and visible emotional responses as a way of recording 'evidence' of instantaneous wellbeing benefits had proved very useful in the earlier interventions at the nursing home on Merseyside.

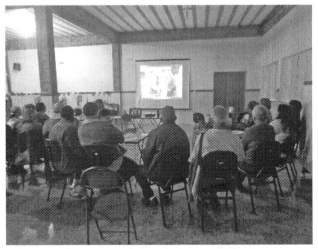

Fig. 1.1. Watching Old Movie Clips at Fazenda Inglesa GP Practice.

The audience also participated in other ludic activities, such as having their photographs taken 'dressed' as one of two famous stars – Carmen Miranda for the ladies, and Mazzaropi, a famous Brazilian male comedian, for the gentlemen. This feat was simply achieved by commissioning a local amateur artist to create fairground-style 'aunt sallies' reproducing the familiar costumes of these two stars of Brazilian cinema (see Fig. 1.2).

FEEDBACK AND RESULTS

The GP and the team of six ACSs played a vital role in selecting the participants and in supporting their involvement in the event. Afterwards the participants completed questionnaires – with help from the ACSs where needed – that focussed on possible benefits of the event in terms of their

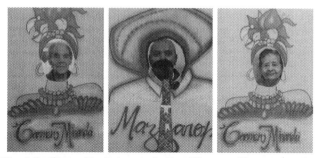

Fig. 1.2. Three Participants in the *Cinema, Memory and Wellbeing* Event at the Fazenda Inglesa GP Practice, Maria José dos Santos (on the Left), Gecilio Donato de Almeida (in the Middle) and Maria de Freitas e Silva (on the Right).

wellbeing. They were invited to provide additional feedback, and the following comments, among many others in a similar vein, were made:

'Sensational! I felt like I travelled through time';

'Having this experience with my neighbours, and feeling that they were also carried away by the emotion of their memories, left me very happy';

'Afterwards I felt much better and livelier';

'This gives older people encouragement to overcome certain things';

'It reawakened my emotional memory of a distant past';

'A benefit was that it distracted me, making me forget the problems at home'.

Lisa interviewed the ACS team after the event, and one of them summarized the positive benefits as follows: 'It brought the participants, friends, health professionals and colleagues together. Throughout the event happiness was stamped in the bright eyes and gestures of all those involved.' Lisa conducted follow-up interviews with the ACS team two months later, and obtained the following important testimony from one of the team:

> *As a result of the event, my view of the old people changed – I discovered that they need more attention, company, affection, more activities specifically for them. There was one man who was very reserved and shy. Since the cinema event he hugs and kisses us and his shyness has disappeared, thanks to our display of affection. He has become more talkative, more active and more hopeful – he keeps asking when we are going to do an event of that kind again. Before one old man didn't want to go but he really enjoyed the event. On the day of the event my grandmother didn't want to go, but she also really enjoyed it and is always asking when the next event will be. They are all asking when the next event will be. One man who took part is now bed-ridden but insists he is going to the next cinema event. Before the public had a more formal relationship with us (the ACS team) – but after seeing us in fancy dress (see Fig. 1.3) they are now more at ease with us, more willing to talk and open up to us. It has helped to break down the barriers between us and the patients. They now invite all of us (ACS team) to go into their home (before the event they wouldn't let us in, and we dealt with them on the doorstep).*

This same ACS added:

> *I was actually thinking of leaving the profession but after the event I had second thoughts, as I realised my job was worthwhile and that I was needed. I felt more valued. In our team we became closer*

> *afterwards, even with difficult colleagues. We no*
> *longer think in terms of our individual 'micro-area'*
> *or 'our old people' – we now have a sense that we are*
> *all in this together, a team.*

An unexpected benefit was the positive impact on the ACS team, who are paid the minimum wage and generally feel undervalued. Another commented that 'the event made me more motivated about my job. It gave us more ideas. We're now thinking of other events to do this year, and the team morale as a whole improved a lot', and another added: 'I was very happy with the participation of the entire team, our coming together was gratifying'. Another ACS, initially very reluctant to become involved in the project, gave the following positive testimony:

> *This project with the older people was a surprising*
> *and gratifying experience. Surprising because, at*
> *first, I thought it didn't make any sense; to be*
> *honest, I thought it was silly. But when it started,*
> *even before the film presentation was screened,*
> *when we visited the old people at home to invite*
> *them and get their consent, my view changed*
> *entirely. On one of these visits I went with Lisa and*
> *two other ACSs, and I saw how the old people felt*
> *important at being invited to the event. On the day*
> *of the presentation it was very gratifying to see them*
> *all. They were excited, they enjoyed themselves and*
> *they re-lived moments from their past life intensely.*

Lisa interviewed the GP two months after the event and he gave the following detailed testimony, highlighting the positive benefits of the initiative for his patients:

> *The* Cinema, Memory and Wellbeing *project can be*
> *considered as an innovative initiative in the context*

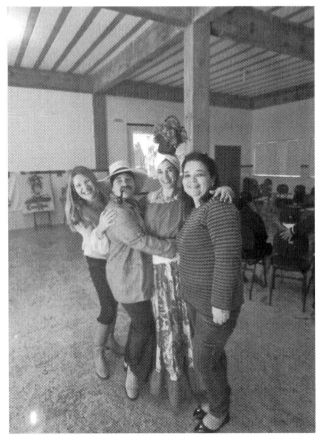

Fig. 1.3. Lisa Shaw (Far Left) with Three of the ACSs from the Fazenda Inglesa GP Practice (From left to right Ana Beatriz [Bia] dos Santos Renter Molter, Zélia de Fátima de Souza and Lilian Pereira Amaral Sá). Bia and Zélia are dressed as the popular Brazilian film stars Mazzaropi and Carmen Miranda, respectively.

of PICS (Integrative and Complementary Health Practices), where the entire team participates, bringing them into closer contact with end users and the end users coming into closer contact with each other. The project can be adapted to suit the local culture, and has a simple methodology, needing only an appropriate physical space, preparation of the venue and the good will and understanding of the participants. The equipment, transport and refreshments for the events are low cost, and this can be covered by management interested in promoting this beneficial activity. The target audience is the older population, who can be included in the activity regardless of whether the individual concerned has a physical or mental illness, provided that s/he is assisted and made comfortable by the entire team. The aim of the project, via the screening of scenes selected from films of an earlier era, is to evoke reminiscences and stimulate within the group the sharing of personal experiences from that era. Via the selection of images, humorous scenes, dialogues using simple language and musical numbers, the participants experience feelings of nostalgia. Even those who at the beginning were sleepy and shy are stimulated by the scenes and the brief interruptions for questions and comments made by the event leader, then joining in with those who are already feeling enthusiastic. We know that it is very common for older people to talk about the past, saying 'in my day' or 'in my youth' it was like this or that, for example. Screening films from an earlier era embraces such discourse, instead of prejudicially viewing it as outdated and fossilised. We are therefore meeting the need of older people to talk about their experiences and establish contact with their historical identity rather than our tendency to withhold their past. Since this is not an invasive *research experiment, we did not use electronic sensors to detect synaptic neuroplasticity in the participants' brains. We relied solely on their oral and physical responses during and after the activity. During the four events organised by the Team, I observed a wealth of physiognomies, reactions and surprising oral accounts. I also felt involved in the 'transtemporality' that this group event provides, revisiting some sensations from childhood.*

The GP's comments also acknowledged how the event had positive outcomes for his own professional role:

I was very happy to take part in the project, extending my activities beyond the mere doctor-patient relationship to embrace interactions with them [the patients] in a context of socialising and research. As I filmed the audience during over 8 hours of projections, as their reactions, comments and emotions unfolded, I was able to see aspects of each individual via their physiognomy. I could never obtain such information in the confines of the consultation room. In the second part of the project, the participants told me a lot about how important meeting up with their neighbours, with whom they have little contact, had been. Some of them revealed that they felt isolated, sad and lacking in stimulation, and that this activity had re-invigorated their lives, making them happier. They spontaneously reported that their mood and behaviour had improved during and after the film screenings, leading me to believe that this type of activity can provide neuro-sensory stimuli, reactivating dormant areas, and reshaping connections in the brain.

The results of the project at the Fazenda Inglesa practice were presented in the form of a poster at the 23rd annual research week (*Semana Científica*) at the Faculty of Medicine in Petrópolis (Faculdade Arthur Sá Earp, 24–27 October 2017) by the practice nurse. The results were summarized as follows: '68 older people took part in the project and were fully involved in the activities. Only one left the session midway through due to feeling unwell. Some of them became animated at seeing clips of old films and many seemed to be very happy during the event.' The poster concluded that 'such activities that promote wellbeing through social events with a cultural focus should be prioritized by Primary Care teams given the few initiatives aimed at the older population and the benefits that such activities can generate.' As a spontaneous initiative designed as a 'thank you' to send to Lisa, who was by now back in Liverpool, one of the ACS team made a short film in July 2015 interviewing some of those who had attended the *Cinema, Memory and Wellbeing* event in April of that year. The following is a transcript of some of sections of the interviews:

Gentleman 1: 'For me it was excellent. It was fun. For us it was a very big incentive. It was very good. I hope it happens again. It was very worthwhile.'

Gentleman 2: 'I was really looking forward to it. I enjoyed it a lot.'

Lady 1 (his wife): 'He was like a child. He wanted to dress like Mazzaropi [Brazilian comic star]' [laughs]

Lady 2: 'Lisa, I loved your idea. The get-together was very good, very educational. […] They were good memories you gave me. I remembered lots of things. And I laughed a lot. I thought it was a sensational idea.'

Lady 3: 'It made me very happy. I send you a big hug, [Lisa]'.

Gentleman 3: 'I loved the cinema event. Next time I want to go again.'

Lady 4: 'It was great [the event] with *Dona* Lisa. A hug and kiss for her!'

Gentleman 4: 'I liked the event a lot. It was marvellous. We met up with friends. If they do it again, I'll go again.'

Lady 5: 'It relaxed us. We felt good. Everyone [was] happy, cheerful. If it happens again, we'll go again.'

Gentleman 5: 'For me all initiatives related to preserving memory are absolutely important and necessary. From a personal point of view seeing images from films that populated my youth [...] was a very special gift. Those images populated our imaginary. Where I lived in Ramos there were lots of cinemas, three cinemas, we went a lot, there was no television. Cinema was our great language. [...] The *chanchadas* [musical comedy films] represent a little of how Brazil was at that moment. Furthermore, having that experience with people, neighbours, from here in Rocio, and feeling that they were moved by their memories made me very happy. I'd like to congratulate the researcher and all the team. I hope this project continues.'

DEVELOPING THE 'BEST-PRACTICE' TOOLKIT

At the end of this first phase of the project, we undertook a qualitative analysis of the materials, including the video evidence, recorded interviews and chats with participants and staff, as well as the questionnaires. We had ample evidence to convince ourselves that the screenings had yielded the following benefits:

For the participants:

- Stimulation of memory and a sensation of emotional wellbeing via reminiscence;

- Generation of a sensation of collective wellbeing via group activities and exchanges of reminiscences and life experiences;

- Improvements in confidence, self-esteem, sociability and mood;

- Reduction of social isolation and feelings of loneliness;

- Reduction of anxiety and depression, albeit perhaps only temporary;

- Focus on wellbeing and prevention of illnesses, both physical and mental (emotional benefits).

For health professional and carers:

- Strengthening of links with the community and within the health-care team;

- Two-way improvements in the relationship between the health workers and their patients;

- Acquisition of new skills and ideas;

- Improvements in wellbeing of the individual and greater work satisfaction.

Given this very positive set of outcomes, we set about designing a 'best-practice' toolkit that would enable healthcare managers and their co-workers, assistants and volunteers to stage their own *Cinema, Memory and Wellbeing* events, using materials and equipment that are readily available in many care homes and day centres. Our main concerns were to ensure that the toolkit was easy to understand and use, that issues of copyright would not stand in the way of the screenings and that it would be engaging enough to encourage people to have fun designing their own *Cinema, Memory and Wellbeing* events. To encourage people to use the toolkit, we decided to include a DVD of film clips featuring local scenes from the 1950s organized by theme; this would enable staff to set up a session without having to worry about finding material if there was difficulty accessing an Internet connection or insufficient broadband width to download material. We were impressed by the range of DVD resources offered by the Yorkshire Film Archive that provide an in-depth focus on specific topics over time, such as holidays and working life, but we wanted a collection of clips that would engage both women and men across a wide range of activities and working situations from a specific time period, as this had worked well with participants at the nursing home. Using her knowledge of films made in and about Liverpool in the 1950s, Julia obtained copyright clearance to create a 10-minute series of clips, and North West Film Archive provided the expertise to create the DVD from their archive materials. The clips are presented as DVD chapters; each clip can be presented independently, allowing time for interaction between the presenter and the group. We decided not to have a soundtrack, thus allowing the presenter to give general pointers and prompts based on each theme and encouraging participants to comment on and engage with the material.

The toolkit is designed as a set of laminated cards, held together by a ring that can be used to hang them on a hook in an office or alongside a TV set/DVD player. The first part of the toolkit makes the case for holding an event, with photographs and quotes from previous participants (useful if anyone needs to argue for additional funding or other kinds of support for an event). The separate, detachable cards mean that presenters can choose which pages they wish to refer to during the event, and in which order, using them as prompt cards where necessary. The toolkit includes a clear explanation of the role of the presenter (page 12) and a checklist for the equipment that is needed (page 10). Pages 13–16 have a list of potential questions about each of the clips for those using the attached DVD 'Liverpool in the 1950s', and page 17 features general questions that could be asked about any clips that could be screened from YouTube or similar online sources. On page 18 there are various suggestions for additional activities that could accompany a film event, such as making posters or simple costumes or hats, or creating a quiz to accompany the clips. Finally, there is a list of useful online resources, providing access to photographs, films and other information about Liverpool. The toolkit was piloted by care homes in Liverpool during 2017 and in Brazil in 2019, the results of which we discuss in detail in Chapter 3.

PARTNERSHIP WITH COMPANY MATTERS4U DAY-CARE CENTRES, LIVERPOOL

[This project is] enabling people to flourish in the 3rd Age (Eleanor O'Hanlon, company director of Company Matters4U day-care centres)

Company Matters4U was set up in 2017 by Debra Murphy and Eleanor (Ellie) O'Hanlon to help tackle social isolation for older people in Liverpool by running day-centre-based activities for people with personal care problems and/or early onset memory loss. In September 2017 we held three *Cinema, Memory and Wellbeing* events at Company Matters4U's day-care centre at Middleton Court in Speke, Liverpool, which were attended by a total of 60 older people. For this project, we decided to focus more intently on recreating the cinema-going experience. We enlisted the help of our friend and colleague from the Department of Music at the University of Liverpool, Professor Sara Cohen, to provide the added attraction of a 1950s musical soundtrack that would play while the audience took their seats and during the interval. We had already established that the running order of the programme worked well – showing the 'newsreel-type' documentary clips first, followed by an interval and then the 'main feature' of clips from a range of Hollywood musical comedies starring Carmen Miranda. We added a portable digital speaker to our technical kit to improve the sound, made sure that the room was as dark as possible and commandeered our wonderful hosts, Ellie and Debra, to dress up as usherettes and serve retro-style refreshments in the interval such as ice creams in wafer sandwiches and boiled sweets from decorated trays they had made from fruit boxes (see Fig. 1.4).

In the first half of the film presentation, the audience clearly took great delight in recognizing and commenting on images of old Liverpool, identifying locations associated with their younger lives, and sharing reminiscences with each other. The following phrases are just a few examples:

'Oh! I remember walking down those steps with my mother!'

'I remember walking through bombed out houses!'

'My brother had a stall on the old [St. John's] market. ...
There was a woman selling flowers – a couple of them. We all used to go there for flowers'

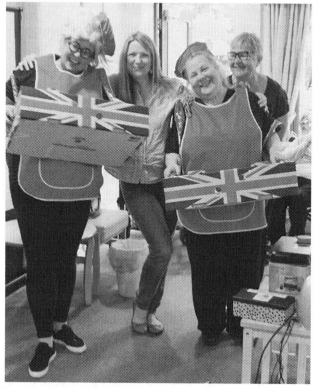

Fig. 1.4. Eleanor [Ellie] O'Hanlon, Lisa Shaw, Debra Murphy and Julia Hallam (Left to Right) at the *Cinema, Memory and Wellbeing* Event at a Company Matters4U Day-care Centre in Liverpool.

'I used to work in that Co-op. I served Bessie Braddock once! I was about 20 or 22'

'I used to travel on the Overhead Railway. I worked at Tate & Lyle's'

'You used to get stuck in them tram lines with your bike wheels!'

Archival footage of various workplaces in Liverpool elicited
animated interjections, including the following:

'I worked at Evans Medical for 12 years. I was in the office,
taking samples to the lab. I enjoyed it.'

'I used to be a conductress on the trams. [...] The 26, which
used to do Princes Road, and the 14, Utting Avenue'

'I worked at Jacob's, me. I used to get the kids ready for
school, 6 kids. [...] Jacob's factory – biscuits, crackers. Long
Lane. Jam works right opposite. [...] I did the boxes.
Sometimes they put me in the chocolate room, where the
chocolate was. I was made up! You could eat as many as
you wanted, but if they found any in your bag you got
sacked.'

Several women discovered they had all previously worked
on the production line at the local Dunlop factory, and carried
on chatting long after the session had finished. One of them
declared: 'I made golf balls there. [...] My mum used to say
"Get some wellies for the kids", my brothers. You had to pay
but got them cheap.'

Location shots of war-damaged buildings and bomb sites
provoked a rich exchange of memories relating to the Second
World War, which captured a child's sense of adventure
rather than any traumatic reactions. One man laughed as he
remembered the following: 'When the railway got bombed,
we lived at the back of that. [...] I don't really remember 'cos I
slept through it.' Another recalled that when there was an air
raid 'we'd go into the cellar. ... I remember bits of shrapnel on
the road, we used to collect it. You have no fear when you're
young. In the next road [a house] got hit and the school got hit
but there was no one in it. [Mum and dad] gave you a crack
over the ear if you did something wrong – Get in here!' He
recalled the air raid warden coming around 'with his gas mask

and his helmet', saying 'Get in the shelter!' He then said: 'There were shelters right outside our house so why we went in the cellar God only knows! [laughs] 7 of us, all cuddling up ... to keep warm.' A couple of women talked about their experiences in the Land Army, another of working for the fire brigade, and a younger woman talked to them about being evacuated aged nine years from Liverpool to Pwllheli in Wales with her cousin: 'We were on the train all day. We got on at West Derby Road. I couldn't get home quick enough. I only stayed about six weeks. [...] We stayed in Northwich about 10 months, but we used to come home at weekends, it was only a bus ride.'

During the interval the audience sang along to some of the hit songs from the 1950s that we played as background music. Most remained seated but swayed or moved their arms to the music, smiling and engaging with each other, but a couple of ladies even asked for help in standing and dancing with us and the care assistants. The musical soundtrack also stimulated a range of comments and interactions, as follows:

'Cilla Black's mother used to work in the indoor market. [...] Her mother was always in the market. Cilla was just singing in little clubs then.'

'Paul McCartney only lived up the road from me.'

'John Lennon's mum lived just opposite me.'

'I liked John more than the others.'

'I wasn't really [a fan]. I was more into Elvis Presley and Gene Pitney.'

For the second part of the show, Lisa introduced the film clips dressed in her Carmen Miranda–inspired carnival costume, passing around images of the star's outlandish costumes, while one of the care assistants, a great dancer, volunteered to put on a spare Miranda outfit and made a 'guest appearance' as the Brazilian star's 'sister' visiting the UK in search of a husband (the gentlemen in the audience loved that one!). The direct involvement of care home staff is extremely important, and the residents/service users gain even greater enjoyment from seeing them singing along with them, dressing up and so on. Our colleague, Sara Cohen, then distributed percussion instruments like maracas and rattles, and members of the audience joined in with the musical numbers enthusiastically, as well as singing along to some of Miranda's more memorable songs. Finally, Julia circulated photocopies of photographs of old cinemas in Liverpool, a technique that had prompted animated discussions at the nursing home. Once again participants were eager to talk about the ones they used to go to. One gentleman recalled: 'We used to go to a little cinema in Liverpool a few footsteps away from the house… The Palladium, it was called. […] In those days I loved the Three Stooges, Curly, Larry and Moe. […] The projector shone over the balcony, you could see cigarette smoke.' When shown several photos of old cinemas in Liverpool, another man said 'I've been to them all. The Futurist, the Palais de Luxe, the Odeon on London Road, and the Trocadero. I used to go mainly on weekends. […] The Warwick … the balcony collapsed in there. I didn't go there that time. The balcony gave way. … I don't think anyone was hurt.' Generating much laughter, a woman then said, when she saw a photo of the Gaumont in the Dingle district: 'I used to go to kiss the lads [in there]'. These interactions led on to others about social life and leisure pursuits in general. One man vividly recalled the following incident at the Rialto ballroom in the city:

> *The Americans, the Yanks from Burtonwood used to go there. There'd be a clash for the girls. The Yanks*

> *against the locals having fights. [...] My brother had*
> *a few black eyes. [...] It was a cinema as well. My*
> *mother went with a couple of my sisters and coming*
> *out it was a black-out and a taxi knocked them*
> *down. Broke my mum's leg.*

Another recounted how he used to go to dances at the Locarno and Grafton ballrooms. 'I was a teddy boy. I used to wear a big long coat and tight trousers'.[4]

The positive benefits for the wellbeing of the participants in the short term were clear to see from the smiles on their faces and the laughter ringing in the air, but longer-term benefits were equally noted by the care workers involved, one of whom remarked that in the weeks that followed some of the shy male members of the audience were more confident in joining in other activities, such as the regular karaoke afternoon; one lady who previously would not sing 'now joins in with gusto'. Another care worker commented: 'Everyone continues to talk about the event and can remember different aspects of the day with positivity and fondness. They are excited and interested in what the next event will be'. To make this 'feel-good' memory last as long as possible, photos taken at the event of audience members in the guise of Charlie Chaplin or Carmen Miranda (poking their heads through

---

4 As part of these discussions about cinema-going, and to assist us in constructing future activities, we asked the audiences who their favourite film stars were: Kirk Douglas, Bette Davies, Grace Kelly, John Wayne, Betty Grable, Audrey Hepburn, Doris Day, Laurel and Hardy, Esther Williams ('a good swimmer!'), Robert Taylor, were all mentioned along with 'Who was that fella in *Gone with the Wind*?' Based on their comments, we are planning film star–themed activities to diversify the content of future events, and to ensure a broad range of engagement across the different tastes and backgrounds of the service users, we will focus on films from a specific period (e.g. 1950–1955), with activities based around, for example, star images, poster design and fashion.

cheaply made, fairground-style 'aunt sallies' of the two stars) were turned into souvenir coasters/small jigsaws – every time they have a cuppa they can remember the fun they had on the day, and share it with the rest of their family and friends.

Ellie O'Hanlon came up with a wonderful phrase to sum up the positive outcomes of the three *Cinema, Memory and Wellbeing* events: 'Enabling people to flourish in the Third Age'. The animated conversations and lively interaction that the film events prompted were captured in a short film made by Pete Carr for the funder of the project, the HOP (Happy Older People) Network (National Museums Liverpool/House of Memories/Open Culture/NHS Liverpool Clinical Commissioning Group).[5] One of the care assistants, Rodger Moire, celebrated the sessions with a specially composed poem that now features on the back page of the final version of the toolkit. Ellie O'Hanlon wrote in her feedback on the events: 'Service users quite enjoyed the one-on-one attention (photo opportunities, use of props/costumes). They enjoyed sharing their memories and experiences with each other and with the hosts.' An unexpected benefit for staff was the way it broke down barriers, enabling new employees, in particular, to connect with service users on a more personal level. O'Hanlon stated:

> *This event took place at the beginning of the new service and was an excellent way in which to get to know the service users (for the staff team). Service users said that it was different to anything that they had done before at the centre and was fun and relaxing. They took great delight in recognising*

---

5 The HOP film can be accessed here: https://happyolderpeople.com/about/hop-pot-small-grants/. The last three minutes of the film cover some of our project work in Speke, Merseyside. You can access a longer version here: https://stream.liv.ac.uk/rk9rrrb9.

> *images of old Liverpool and this promoted lots of*
> *positive discussion. Seeing the service users' reaction*
> *to the event, we were then able to build on that and*
> *come up with individual strategies for enabling*
> *individuals to get the most from their chosen activity.*

CONCLUSIONS

Perhaps the biggest surprise of the pilot projects as far as we were concerned was the pleasure it brought not only to the participants but also to their carers. All of the people working in the care homes and in the community settings that we worked with went the extra mile to make sure that their service users had a good time, joining in by helping with the paperwork, making and wearing costumes, getting people talking and in some cases, singing and dancing along. This important but often unappreciated group of people, typically working in difficult circumstances with few resources, are the key to ensuring those who can no longer care for themselves continue to enjoy their lives. Given the enthusiasm of the carers and their creativity, we decided to involve them more in co-production of future events, as explored in more details in Chapter 3, broadening the range of activities linked to the screenings to embrace arts and crafts workshops, for example.

The pilot projects left us in no doubt that well-chosen excerpts from actuality footage, documentary and feature films stimulate both individual and collective remembering, and by doing so in a group setting help to combat social isolation. Once one person started recounting a particular story from their memory bank of experiences, others started to join in. This was particularly noticeable amongst the men at Company Matters4U's day-care centre, who tended to be quieter at the sessions at the residential nursing home.

We think this was because the subject matter of the clips, such as motor car racing at Aintree, stone masons working on the completion of the Anglican Cathedral and the loading of huge items such as steam engines onto ships for export at Liverpool's docks, stimulated their interest and their memories, leading to conversations about the nature of their working lives and the often dangerous conditions that they faced at that time. The women too found areas of mutual interest, some of them discovering that they knew relatives who had worked in the same factories, or that they had frequented the same dance halls and cinemas, or that they remembered particular clothing items such as platform-soled shoes. For those who were not from Liverpool and had settled in the city, the Carmen Miranda film clips created a shared point of international reference that enabled discussion to focus on music and fashion, connections that we explore more fully in the following chapters. In Chapter 2 we will now look at a pilot project where we focused more closely on the role of music listening in generating positive memories and emotions.

2

MUSIC, MEMORY AND WELLBEING: A PILOT PROJECT IN LIVERPOOL

Jacqueline Waldock and Sara Cohen

INTRODUCTION

Sara Cohen (Professor of Music and Director of the Institute of Popular Music) has a background in social anthropology and has published books, chapters and articles that bring an anthropological approach to the study of popular music. Since the mid-1980s she has carried out research on music's role and significance in the lives of people in England, particularly in the city of Liverpool and the wider Merseyside region. Most of her projects have been conducted in collaboration with various cultural and governmental organizations. They have focussed on musicians, music audiences and music entrepreneurs, and have investigated the musical lives and histories of diverse groups and communities. Among them are projects that have used music as a basis for oral history and reminiscence work with older audiences who frequent local day centres or live in sheltered accommodation for older people. In general, the research for these projects has depended on getting to know the people involved, observing and participating in their music activities, and talking to them about music and what it means to them.

To help elicit people's stories about music and prompt them to remember their musical past, Sara has employed various research methods. They have included inviting people to engage with music objects and items of memorabilia, to draw maps illustrating their musical memories, and to guide her around places of music where they regularly hang out. This research encouraged Sara to reflect on the relationship between music and remembering. Through a number of projects, she has explored how particular communities and organizations engage in a collective remembering of the musical past, as well as how individuals remember their own autobiographical musical past. These projects highlighted music's distinctive influence on how people remember. By providing a soundtrack to people's lives, for example, music becomes associated with experiences that they have accumulated over the years, offering a basis for life mapping. It struck Sara that music could therefore provide a productive and unique focus for research on ageing. By encouraging people to remember the musical past, her recent projects have used this remembering as a lens through which to explore ideas and experiences of age and ageing. They include projects informed by her membership of the international research network 'Ageing, Communication, Technologies' (ACT), and her own personal circumstances as primary carer for her mother, who was living with a progressive neuromuscular disease and dementia diagnosis.[1]

---

1 https://actproject.ca. ACT is an international research and partnership
   project established in 2014 to address the transformation of the experiences
   of ageing with the proliferation of new forms of mediated communications
   in networked societies. The project has been creating intergenerational
   connections, rethinking media from the perspective of old age, and
   confronting ageism.

After moving her mother to a care home, Sara began to explore ways of using her research on music and remembering to enhance the wellbeing of the care home residents, and of others living with dementia or age-related memory loss. Consequently, she participated in the *Cinema, Memory and Wellbeing* events run by Lisa and Julia at the Company Matters4U day-care centre in Speke, Liverpool (Chapter 1), specifically providing musical accompaniments for the interval and talking to the participants about their memories of listening or dancing to music in the city.

Jacky Waldock is a post-doctoral researcher in the Faculty of Humanities and Social Sciences at the University of Liverpool. She has a background in music composition and in community-engaged arts, and has published work on the close relationship between sound and community identity. Her experience of working on community arts projects led her to collaborate with the Foundation for Art and Creative Technology (FACT) on their electric blanket project, which brought digital skills workshops to sheltered housing schemes in Liverpool through creative arts engagement.[2] She has worked in care homes in areas of urban regeneration in Manchester, using music and sound as a tool for talking about spaces that no longer visually exist. Her work has also examined the important role that sound plays in making community and home. This led her to question how people create a sense of community and home through sound as they age, and how age-related illness can break these connections to home and community.

---

2 https://www.fact.co.uk. FACT is a Liverpool-based cinema and art gallery and the UK's leading organization for the support and exhibition of film, art and new media.

In 2018 Sara and Jacky joined forces with Lisa to explore how audio-visual media might be used as a resource for stimulating reminiscence and wellbeing, and for the benefit of those living with dementia and age-related memory loss. The results of this activity are discussed below but with a specific focus on music. First, we review a range of UK music initiatives or 'interventions' targeted at those living with dementia and age-related memory loss. Second, we explain how key projects informed our own approach and work that we are currently undertaking in Liverpool.

MUSIC AND MEMORY INTERVENTIONS IN THE UK

In the UK, the growing number of people aged 65 years and older has intensified the challenge of age-related cognitive decline. This decline affects people's wellbeing and independence, and represents one of the most feared, and economically costly, aspects of ageing. The increasing numbers of those living with it has created new demands for initiatives and merchandise that enable older citizens to lead independent, fulfilled lives, and that attend at the same time to the wellbeing of their families and carers. This has led, among other things, to the emergence of technologies, products, services and activities designed for those living with dementia and age-related memory loss. They include arts-based initiatives and of all of the arts, music has been singled out and celebrated for its unique impact on memory and wellbeing, and as an effective, low-cost contribution to efforts to tackle the 'problem' of ageing. According to the 2018 Commission on Dementia and Music, for example, 'music offers a potential lifeline for people with dementia, their carers and loved ones, one which can sometimes be unmatched by other interventions'.[3]

This emphasis on music is supported by research that has explored the potential cognitive, social and psychological wellbeing benefits of musical experience for older adults. Music psychologists have documented a positive association between musical experience and cognitive abilities (see, for example, Osman, Tischler, & Schneider, 2016), while observational and interventionist research conducted with older adults has highlighted the role of listening to music, singing or playing a musical instrument in managing symptoms of depression or anxiety, and promoting psychological wellbeing (Costa, Ockelford, & Hargreaves, 2018). A 2019 report by the International Longevity Centre UK (ILC) and the Utley Foundation found that music has significant physical and mental health benefits for those with dementia, and helps them to retain their speech and language skills for a longer period of time: 'Analysis showed that music helps to significantly minimise some of the symptoms of dementia, such as agitation, and can help to tackle anxiety and depression'. (Sally Greengross, chief executive of the ILC).

In the Introduction, we mentioned the US documentary *Alive Inside: A Story of Music and Memory* (2014), which featured the renowned neurologist Oliver Sacks and was key in bringing dementia and the benefits of music to a wider public. The film follows the wondrous effect of personalized music on those living with dementia. One scene, for example, features a care home resident who, according to her carer, did not open her eyes or speak until the moment they played music for her, and she then

---

3 http://www.ilcuk.org.uk/index.php/news/news_posts/press_release_new_
   commission_brings_evidence_based_research_and_recommendations.

started shaking her feet and moving her head to its rhythm. The film also shows how hearing music sparked the reminiscences of others living with dementia, as well as singing and dancing. The film received the audience award at the 2014 Sundance Film Festival and since then has gone on to be aired in Norway, Britain, France, Estonia, Brazil and other countries. The heightened awareness of music's benefits for wellbeing that it garnered helped to encourage central government support for a wide range of social prescribing activities in the UK. As we noted in the Introduction, social prescribing refers to the promotion/ recommendation of activities that bring people together and enable wellbeing. As well as community groups and walking groups, social prescribing embraces the promotion of music-related activities such as choirs. 'Singing should be on prescription', states Grenville Jones, founder of the Golden Oldies charity, which uses collective singing to bring people together and reduce isolation and loneliness.[4] In 2018 the UK Government's Health and Wellbeing Fund awarded £4.5 million to 23 social prescribing projects, which led to funding for social prescribing link workers based within NHS trusts to be funded in 2019.

Beyond the established, professional practice of Music Therapy, therefore, music has been incorporated into strategies for promoting 'healthy ageing'. This has involved a broad range of 'interventions', a term that has been used to describe intentional music-based activities in therapeutic or care-based settings, whether karaoke, singing or music-making sessions, or reminiscence workshops. These activities are delivered by a multiplicity of practitioners, from musicians, entertainers and choir masters, to groups and

---

4 http://www.golden-oldies.org.uk.

organizations across the public, private, community and voluntary sectors.

Focussing on a few specific interventions, the following discussion illustrates some of the diverse ways in which music has provided a basis for initiatives targeted at those living with dementia/memory 'loss'. The best-known and most celebrated interventions are those based on live music. We consider how live music performances of various kinds are commonly used to improve the wellbeing of people who are being cared for in residential or private homes, whether as entertainment, as a mechanism for social participation or as a memory prompt. One of our main arguments, however, is that music does not have to be performed live in order to achieve such effects, so we end our review of UK music interventions by discussing those involving digital and recorded music.

SINGING FOR THE BRAIN

The choral organization *Singing for the Brain* came to the public's attention through the BBC documentary *Our Dementia Choir with Vicky McClure* (2019). Established by the UK's Alzheimer's Society in 2003, the organization's aims are:

- To improve and maintain neurological pathways through gentle aerobic activity.

- To help carers and persons with dementia see each other in happy circumstances where both have been stimulated to enjoy communication.

- To lift or prevent depression through the use of elements which will surprise, reassure, support, inspire and mediate reframing a negative life viewpoint into a positive one.

- To become something General Practitioners can recommend to patients, as they do [physical] exercise, and thus help them to feel diagnosis is worth doing.

- To help families with dementia 'come out' and feel part of society where they have a right to artistic and social stimulation.

- To encourage carers and people with dementia to be proactive in looking after themselves, to network with others in the same boat who might exchange help.

- To give families a view of themselves as managers of their life not victims of fate. (Bamford & Clift, 2007, p. 7)

Singing for the Brain sessions involve several elements, including coffee and chatting, singing and movement. The song choices in the sessions have specific purposes:

- To enforce the importance of the individual in the group, and integrate people into the singing community, through a 'welcome song' that introduces and welcomes each person by name.

- To strengthen co-ordination and aerobic activity through movement.

- To support reminiscence through the singing of familiar songs from the past.

In *Singing for the Brain* sessions the music acts as a prompt for discussion of past experiences and events within a group setting. However, as we can see from the above list, the aims of *Singing for the Brain* go beyond reminiscence and are designed to also foster 'social interactions, peer support, engagement and active participation to improve quality of life' (Osman et al., 2016). The way these sessions support and encourage those living with dementia and their carers to attend an activity is beneficial in and of itself, helping to diminish apathy and isolation for both groups.

ORCHESTRAS REACH OUT

Over the past decade several of the UK's leading orchestras have taken an active role in making their programmes more accessible to people from a wide range of backgrounds. One prominent development is the establishment of dementia-friendly concerts and concert spaces. These concerts are often focussed around those living with dementia and have been built on the back of both research into, and public awareness of, the significance of music for memory. In 2018 the disability-led charity Attitude is Everything granted its top 'gold status' award to the Liverpool Philharmonic Orchestra for its disability-friendly provision that includes Relaxed and Dementia-Friendly Concerts.[5] Along with several other orchestras, the Liverpool Philharmonic has also moved beyond the staging of dementia-friendly concerts within the concert hall, by sending musicians to meet with care providers and service users in hospitals, care homes and supported living settings. In doing so, they have created safe spaces in which those living with dementia can access music, while also devising innovative approaches to music-making.[6] Through these approaches they have sought to harness music's impact on people's emotions, social relationships and participation, thereby seeking to enrich the lives of those living with dementia and their carers.

5 https://www.liverpoolphil.com/plan-your-visit/accessibility/attitude-is-everything/.

6 https://www.liverpoolphil.com/about-us/.

The outreach programmes of the City of Birmingham Symphony Orchestra, the Hallé Orchestra and the London Symphony Orchestra (LSO) help to illustrate this trend. The City of Birmingham Symphony Orchestra gave its first concert in 1920 and now performs over 150 concerts a year across a wide range of musical styles. Alongside this extensive concert schedule, the orchestra runs a number of community-based activities, including chamber music performances staged in retirement villages run by ExtraCare, a charitable trust that operates in the Midlands and aims to provide 'better lives for older people'.[7] The Orchestra also works specifically with those living with dementia through weekly visits by four of its musicians to care homes in Birmingham, where they run music workshops. These workshops are not based around musicians performing pieces *for* the care home residents. Rather, the residents and their carers are instead encouraged to participate *in* the musical performance, contributing sounds and ideas through rhythms, discussion and instrumental noise-making. In this sense they are workshops based on music improvisation. Unlike the dementia-friendly concerts where the onus on the concertgoers is to listen to and enjoy the music, these workshops involve musicians working with the care home residents to collectively create new musical works as the music is being performed.

The improvisation workshops run by musicians from the City of Birmingham Symphony Orchestra are in some ways similar to those run by music therapists. According to the Canadian Association for Music Therapy (CAMT), 'Music has nonverbal, creative, structural and emotional qualities. These are used in therapeutic relationships to facilitate contact, interaction, self-awareness, learning, self-expression, communication and personal development'. The therapeutic

---

7 https://www.extracare.org.uk/about-the-charity/the-trust-overview/.

aspects of the City of Birmingham Symphony Orchestra workshops are highlighted by comments made by the orchestra's cellist Jackie Tyler: 'The workshops are all about nonverbal communication and human interaction, which we simulate through music-making in a shared and incredibly supportive environment'.[8] Here, the purpose of the music sessions and the role of the musicians is not to trigger reminiscence in the residences through musical listening. Rather, they are producing new works that support the participants' personal and creative experiences, enabling the music to be a source for personal expression, leadership and social interaction without the need for verbal communication. Jackie Tyler's comments show how the workshops are about human interaction and the forging of social relationships between people who come together to create a piece of music. Consequently, the music-making supports a sense of 'we-ness', a concept that was discussed in the Introduction, and of connection between and among the service users and the musicians, thereby allowing for a creation of community and belonging.

The Hallé Orchestra is one of the oldest orchestras in the UK and performed its first concert in 1858. The orchestra performs a wide range of music and over 110 concerts a year, staged in Manchester and across the country. It also runs several activities that reach beyond the bounds of the concert hall, including tea dances, a scheme that teaches inmates at the correctional facility HMP Thorn Cross to play brass instruments, and a specialist strand of work entitled 'Care in the Community'. This latter strand includes a Musician-in-Residence project with the Pendine Park care home in Wrexham. This project predominantly works as an enrichment programme that seeks to improve the quality of life for all

---

8 https://cbso.co.uk/news/music-for-wellbeing.

residents of the home and particularly those with dementia. The Hallé's musicians work with residents in a responsive way to create music. This involves the musicians taking visual cues from the residents, such as hand gestures and the tapping of fingers, or arm and eye movements, and using them as instructions that inform their performance and the piece of music they create.

The approach of the Hallé is similar to that taken by the City of Birmingham Symphony Orchestra, where the music is created *with* the residents rather than solely performed *to* them. However, the use of these visual cues as a guide for music-making distinguishes the Hallé approach, with the orchestra's musicians not just performing the music but also taking on the role of composer and conductor.[9] The Hallé orchestra's partnership with the Pendine Park care home also enables the orchestra to explore how technology can improve the relationship between service users and musicians.[10] This has led to the employment of a technology called MYO at the workshops, including the MYO armband. This armband reads movement in the arm by registering electroactivity, turning small muscle movements that may not be clearly visible into sounds, so that residents with limited or restricted movement are nevertheless able to participate in the music-making process. The use of this type of technology is new and relatively limited. In videos produced by the Hallé, the armbands were attached to tubes or cushions and utilized as a digital sound-making device, rather than being used on the body.[11] It is hoped that in the future these devices may be

9   https://www.halle.co.uk/education/community-projects/work-with-older-people/.

10 http://pendinepark.com/news-pioneering-arts-training.html.

11 https://www.youtube.com/watch?v=os6Q0EDbkK0.

developed in thoughtful and meaningful ways to allow a widening participation in music composition.

The LSO runs an extensive programme of 'accessible' activities. They include informal lunchtime concerts and regular hospital visits undertaken by the orchestra's musicians to the Newham University, Whipps Cross and Royal London hospitals. These hospital visits are organized in partnership with Vital Arts, a charitable organization that uses the arts, including music workshops, to improve patients' experience in hospital settings.[12] Vital Arts was founded in 1996 to 'Deliver arts project that enhance the hospital environment and, in turn, improve the patient experience'. The organization's aim is to provide 'meaningful cultural encounters which they [the patients] might not otherwise access'. Its work extends beyond classical music, incorporating world music and other art forms into the hospital experience, including dance and visual arts interventions.

At Newham University Hospital, the LSO provides musicians and a workshop leader who support patients in five Older Adult Wards. This work is assisted by the hospital's Dementia and Delirium team. Although these wards are not exclusively dementia wards, 60% of the patients receiving treatment on the wards are living with some form of dementia.[13] The LSO's approach is to provide a participatory as well as a performance experience, and in this setting the experience of both musicians and audiences is vastly different from that of the formal concert hall. Classical concert halls are traditionally places for quiet contemplation and concentrated listening. The noise-making of the concert hall audiences is usually limited to clapping at the end of a

---

12 Vital Arts is the arts organization for Barts Health NHS Trust, the largest Trust in the UK.

13 https://lso.co.uk/lso-discovery/community/hospital-visits.html.

piece or perhaps the stamping of feet if the response is particularly effusive. However, by working alongside workshop leaders and health care specialists in hospital settings, the LSO musicians have enabled musical experiences that are less formal and constrained, without compromising the excellence of the musicianship or the quality of the performance. The hospital workshops often include vocal warm-ups and encourage all of the participants to engage with the music through singing, playing or dancing. This environment allows the patients involved to talk to the musicians and be in close proximity to them as they perform, thereby building social as well as musical connections.

COMMUNITY AND COMMERCIAL ENGAGEMENT

The live music interventions mentioned so far highlight the role that music can play in bringing people together. It enables them not only to establish social relationships but also to develop a sense of connection and collective identity. This connective-ness (the 'we-ness' discussed in the Introduction, p. 29) is not limited to official, high-profile initiatives or to those that are therapy-led, such as *Singing for the Brain* or the outreach work of professional orchestral players. It is also enabled through live music initiatives delivered by numerous grass-roots organizations, including community and voluntary groups, and by individuals, groups and organizations operating across the commercial sector. At the care home where Sara's mother resides, for example, local school pupils have visited once or twice to sing to the care home residents, and a professional singer visits on a monthly basis to perform classic popular songs from the 1950s and 1960s. This is not an easy audience to perform to, since audience members often have to move (with or without help) around and out of the room for reasons that have little to do with the musical performance, and not all of them are able to respond to it. Usually, however, the performance elicits singing or even dancing, and a sense of connection and participation that can be strongly felt.

The benefits of such performances for care home residents, most of them in their 80s and older, are highlighted by specialist agents, such as Care Home Entertainers UK, Musicteam, and Full Beam Productions. These agents provide entertainment for various organizations that cater for older people and those living with dementia and age-related memory loss. Operating under the banner 'the future of care home entertainment', Full Beam Productions emphasizes the importance of giving residents a choice in terms of the music that is played, and encourages care homes to submit their requests one week in advance. They do so partly to counter the assumptions that are commonly made about people's musical tastes, noting that care home residents are not necessarily keen to hear songs that were popular when they were young:

> *Of course, the days of singing Vera Lynn and all of her wartime classics are far from behind us – and I believe that they will always have a firm place in a care home environment, as a way of reminding us of history, and celebrating the fact that we are still here. But [...] we have found an increasing number of residents wanting to hear a few more of their favourite artists from a little later in life.*[14]

Organizations like Making Music provide online support and resources for musicians seeking to perform in care homes,

---

14 https://www.fullbeamproductions.net/care-homes.

and to make them 'more musical places'.[15] So, too, does *A Choir in Every Care Home*, an organization that works in collaboration with organizations from adult social care, music and academic research, as we mentioned in the Introduction.[16] Karaoke events are also commonly used to engage the audiences that such organizations cater for and encourage participation and connectedness, as with the karaoke sessions run by Company Matters4U mentioned in the Introduction to this book. Such events can be specifically designed to prompt reminiscence. The karaoke programmes of The Music Box, for example, are designed by the charity *Sing For Your Life* that works with residential care and nursing homes, hospitals and day-care centres. The Music Box technology is simple to use and does not require any formal musical training to operate. It plugs into a television or can be operated through a projector and speakers. Unlike a typical karaoke machine, the visual and musical backgrounds are relatively simple to avoid confusing audiences (e.g. a one-colour background with only lyrics displayed on it), and the key and speed can be changed to suit the particular group of participants involved. Moreover, images can be shown on the screen – something that the Music Box has found useful for reminiscence purposes.[17]

ENGAGING WITH DIGITAL AND RECORDED MUSIC

The Music Box technology is one of many music technologies and products designed to stimulate music-making, singing and remembering among older audiences, and those living with dementia. There are also commercial music recordings

---

15 https://www.makingmusic.org.uk/membership-and-insurance.

16 http://myhomelife.org.uk/news/music-is-vital-for-care-homes/.

17 http://www.singforyourlife.org.uk/the-silver-song-music-box.

designed for similar purposes, such as albums featuring music hits from particular decades and intended to promote reminiscence and nostalgia. Dementia-friendly music players can also be purchased, such as the Simple Music Player which can be pre-programmed with songs that have been selected and downloaded via a USB link, as can the Unforgettable Music Play that also operates as a radio. There are also dementia-friendly radio stations that commonly broadcast music from the past. One example is Radio Reminisce. Based in Derbyshire, this UK-wide radio station aims to appeal to the network of over 18,000 nursing, residential and care homes across the UK, as well as the many thousands of people living with dementia who are being cared for at home. According to the music publisher James Oldrini who founded the station: 'Radio Reminisce aims to create a community, bring older people together, and get them talking with one another and sharing memories with their carers, family, friends and neighbours.'[18]

Founded in 2013, *Playlist for Life* is likewise keen to help people tap into significant moments from their past through music listening and recorded music. However, unlike the initiatives that have already been discussed, the organization adopts a more personalized approach to music intervention, and advocates headphone listening. During 2019 it featured prominently in a report from the Commission on Dementia and Music, which attracted central government endorsement and extensive coverage in Britain's quality newspapers and on the BBC. The *Playlist for Life* website encourages those living with dementia to create, with the help of their relatives, playlists of musical pieces or songs that have for various reasons played an important part in their lives. It is a simple

---

18 https://nailed.community/2019/05/23/uk-wide-dementia-friendly-radio-launched-by-locals/.

idea and the website provides information and guidance that can help with the creation of these playlists. They include hints and tips on how to search for music using online musical tools such as Spotify and Apple Music, and information on apps that allow people to search for a song by singing a line from it. The organization provides online training to support the use of such playlists in care home settings. Its website lists four ways in which music can be beneficial for listeners, suggesting that it can:

- Bring back feelings, memories and sometimes even abilities thought lost.

- Reduce the use of heavy drugs and restraints.

- Manage mood and emotions.

- Strengthen relationships, reconnect families and support new connections.

More specifically, the website claims that when the playlist is used correctly through 'therapeutic scheduling' and listening sessions that are of 30 minutes' duration, and held before particular activities, it can reduce the use of psychotropic medication, the use of restraints, stress and distress, and wandering.[19]

The playlists are personalized collections of music, similar to what used to be referred to during the 1980s as a 'mix tape'. When explaining the significance of playlists comprising music from the past, the *Playlist for Life* organization refers to 'the memory bump', 'inheritance tracks' and 'identity tracks'.[20] The 'memory bump', or what we

---

19 https://www.playlistforlife.org.uk/the-science.

20 https://www.playlistforlife.org.uk/find-the-right-music.

referred to in the Introduction to this book as a 'reminiscence bump', applies to more easily accessed memories that are formed when individuals were between 12 and 22 years of age. 'Inheritance tracks' are described by *Playlist for Life* as songs or pieces of music that are inherited because they are sung to individuals or learned from people they know. 'Identity tracks' are songs that speak to particular aspects of an individual's identity, such as where they are from.

To help with the creation of playlists by individuals and their relatives or friends, *Playlist for Life* provides a list of questions for them to address:

- Are there any songs or artists linked to childhood? E.g. lullabies or nursery rhymes?

- Are there any wedding songs that could help? E.g. music played at a first dance?

- Can you think of any favourite bands, singers or shows?

- Were there any songs sung at family parties?

- Did you/they enjoy dancing? E.g. classes, disco.

- Could songs from the war conjure any memories?

- Are there TV theme tunes that might stir a memory?

- Are there songs from a holiday?

- Are there favourite Christmas songs?

- Do friends or family have any suggestions?

Playlist for Life does note that music might not always have a positive effect, and that songs that initiate an adverse reaction might need to be marked with a 'red flag':

Music is powerful. It can take you to another time or place. That is a great gift. But you do not want to take someone back to a bad place. If someone becomes very agitated or distressed listening to a certain tune, you should stop the session immediately *and discard that music. Remember that tears on their own are not always bad. They are a sign of deep emotion and sometimes that is an emotion a person would rather have than not. Focus on the person. Are they distressed? If they are not distressed, be with them in that moment. Hold their hand or put an arm round them if it feels appropriate. Spend time with them until the moment has passed. In this way the playlist can become an opportunity for closeness and deeper caring.* (www.playlistforlife.org.uk)

Lisa's work in Brazil (Chapter 1) illustrates this point through the examples of when song performed in films reduced two individuals to tears, as a consequence of the personal memories they evoked. In both cases, the people concerned and their carers wanted to continue participation in the intervention, and stressed how positive this powerful music-triggered reminiscence had been for them.

EXPLORING APPROACHES TO MUSIC AND MEMORY IN LIVERPOOL

Playlist for Life was of particular interest to us because as part of our work with Lisa we were investigating uses of digital and audio-visual media as a resource for stimulating reminiscence and wellbeing. Supported by the University of Liverpool, one of the main aims of this work was to review the growing market in digital tools targeted at personalized, reminiscence-centred wellbeing for older users, including those living with early-stage dementia and their carers. Another aim was to engage with a range of stakeholders, including care providers and tech companies, to identify specific needs and explore aspects of design and accessibility. Given these aims, there were certain aspects of the approach taken by *Playlist for Life* that raised questions for us. One of them concerns unequal access to the online world and digital resources, while another concerns headphone listening and the fact that for audiences over 60 years of age, using such equipment was not necessarily part of their everyday listening experience. The practice of listening to music through headphones became increasingly popular during the 1980s, signifying a shift from shared to individual listening. While *Playlist for Life* can certainly enable older individuals to engage with their own personal, autobiographical music history, we were concerned that the use of headphones and individualized listening might undermine music's effectiveness in enabling social interaction and participation, the sharing of memories and stories, and the development of collective identity ('we-ness').

Consequently, we decided to explore ways of combining the approach of *Playlist for Life* with group-focussed music activities that allow for greater social interaction, much like the live music and music-making activities that we discussed earlier. To help us with this, we partnered up again with Company Matters4U (see Chapter 1) and worked with contacts in their day-care groups at two centres in Liverpool, one based in South Liverpool and the other in the North of the city. We had initially planned to conduct individual sessions with the users to prepare playlists for each of them, but this proved to be impossible due to scheduling constraints. Something else that forced us to be adaptable was the fact that we had been expecting a maximum of 12 people per group but arrived at the first centre to find a group of 25. This group occupied a large, busy and noisy room and we were introduced to the carers as they bustled around it, chatting and going about their usual routine (serving tea, repositioning chairs, helping people in their care to move about, and so on). The second group, whom we visited the following week, was also larger than expected and comprised 20 people.

Members of both groups came from different areas and backgrounds but were generally white, working-class, and over 60 years of age. Most were women from the Liverpool area, and apart from a few friendships within one of the groups, the group members were not familiar with each other. With these initial, exploratory visits, our aim was to encourage members of each group to choose songs from their past that meant something to them, and to create playlists for each centre that were based on people's individual listening histories and preferences. To encourage conversation we had brought with us the 'getting started' questions produced by *Playlist for Life* listed above, while to source the songs that the group members chose we had decided to use YouTube, Spotify and BBC RemArc – the BBC Reminiscence Archive designed to trigger memories and reminiscences in people with dementia. We were keen to play these songs so that the whole group could engage with them, and to record what was said about them.

The first centre we visited had a television that had never been used but we connected it to a computer to give us the option of not only playing music, but also screening music videos from YouTube. YouTube allows users to upload their own videos, which means that a search for the Tom Jones song 'Delilah' might bring up a clip from his 1968 *Top of the Pops* performance, or a cover of the same song by the Tunbridge Wells Ukulele Band. Consequently, while YouTube can be a useful tool for finding a vast array of clips, it is worth checking these clips before selecting one to display on screen. Moreover, songs on YouTube are not necessarily featured as music videos; sometimes, the music is accompanied by still images of the musician(s) or a record sleeve that it is related to. During the sessions that we ran we found that these still images could work just as effectively as videos in prompting conversations, such as those concerning record collections and teenage crushes.

For these sessions we each worked with a group of two to six participants. While we had planned to utilize the 10 *Playlist for Life* questions (referenced above) to kick-start conversations about music and memory, the questions did not elicit the responses we were hoping for and were generally met with silence, so we had to abandon them. Consequently, we tried out alternative ways of encouraging conversation. We referred to our own music memories, for example, in the hope that this would prompt the service users to do likewise, and to local music venues and dance halls that the service users might be familiar with. Whenever a track was mentioned we would search for it online using Spotify or YouTube and play it to the group. Once we began to listen to music together, the conversation flowed more easily, with songs and musical sounds becoming the primary stimuli for remembering and storytelling.

THE CHALLENGES OF MUSIC INTERVENTIONS

Our visits to the two day-care centres presented us with various challenges. For a start, they raised some problems that could have been ironed out in advance. If the care centre visits had not been brought forward, for example, and our original timetable had been adhered to, we would have had time to conduct one-to-one sessions with each user of the centre and prepare a playlist for them before working with them in groups. The visits nevertheless presented us with challenges that were helpful in a couple of respects: firstly, they raised various questions and concerns about the music initiatives that we reviewed earlier in this chapter, as will become clear in the discussion below; secondly, they highlighted several important issues that should be addressed as part of any initiative targeted at music, reminiscence and wellbeing, and the discussion below focusses on those concerning expectation, setting, cognitive ability and technology.

In terms of expectation, with any initiative or intervention targeted at reminiscence and wellbeing, it is important that the aims are clarified and agreed at an early stage by those participating. In our case, the participants included the service users, their carers, and us – the researchers. For us, the care centre visits were an opportunity to test out particular ways of using music to engage older audiences and enable remembering and wellbeing. While this was explained to the other participants, it was clear that for them, the visits also offered a diversion from their usual weekly routine and the promise of some musical entertainment. Occasionally, these expectations competed with each other. During the second workshop, for example, Miriam selected the song 'A Spaceman Came Travelling' released in 1990 by Chris de Burgh. She chose it because it was a favourite of her late husband and he used to sing it all the time, and it was one of the more recent songs chosen by the group members. At the same time, however, it was less familiar than most of the other songs they chose and not as upbeat. Many of the songs had prompted spontaneous singing as they were played but this Chris de Burgh song brought about a change in mood, so much so that the carers asked us to play something else. On its website, *Playlist for Life* states that music can trigger memories, lift moods and build relationships. In our experience, however, encouraging people to connect music with their autobiographical memories did not necessarily lift their mood or enable the building of relationships between the people in the room. Given that we were working with groups rather than individuals, this example also raises the question of how to cater for both individual and group interests or preferences.

The setting for music initiatives and events is another important issue to consider. The physical setting, for example, has an impact on what happens in these events, and might include factors such as the size, layout and furnishing of the spaces in which these events take place. This same issue is highlighted by Gray, Evans, Griffiths, and Schneider (2017), a group of scholars who specialize in dementia studies and music psychology. In a journal article that reflects critically on the methodological challenges of arts and dementia evaluation and research (2017), these scholars highlight the importance of the spaces in which arts activities are staged and experienced. At both of the day-care centres we visited, our music sessions took place in a large room with a kitchen attached to it. They were multi-purpose rooms – spaces where people could sit at tables and eat lunch or tea, gather together for a workshop or group activity of some kind, or spend the time alone or in smaller groups at the outer edges of the room. We had to contend, therefore, with the clatter of cups and plates emanating from the kitchen, and the continual movement of the workshop participants as carers helped people to move from one chair to another, or to leave the room for a comfort break. This made it difficult for us to engage all of the group members at the same time and encourage social integration. On the other hand, it allowed those who were less willing to engage to opt out of the collective singing and discussion, yet remain in the same social space.

Knowledge of the cognitive, and to a lesser extent physical abilities of the participants, is another important factor. It was clear that there was a multiplicity of cognitive abilities amongst the groups involved in our sessions:

- There were participants who understood the questions being asked and had memories and ideas to share but lacked the physical ability to express them.

- There were participants who understood the terms of the questions but found aspects of them difficult to grasp or process. They could not distinguish yesterday from 10 years ago, for example, and were therefore unable to cope with concepts such as 'memory' or 'the past', and to produce appropriate or articulate responses.

- There were participants who could not understand the questions we asked because they were unable to process the words we used and make them meaningful. The questions therefore became insignificant.

As we tried to accommodate and cater for these various responses and needs, the support we received from carers and family members was invaluable. This was particularly the case with the first group we engaged with. Some of the group members had been meeting together for a while, so friendships had been established between a few of them and the carers and group facilitators were familiar to them. The facilitators had arranged for several family members to join the group to support us in asking questions and encouraging conversation. This helped us to navigate the differing cognitive impairments that existed amongst the group. The second group was based in a North Liverpool centre that was quite new, so its users had not been meeting together for very long, they did not have any family members with them and the carers did not know them particularly well. Consequently, it was harder to navigate the differing cognitive abilities of those within this group since the carers were less familiar with the group members, and we lacked the kind of vital knowledge that family members had brought to the first group.

Technology is another issue that has to be addressed as part of initiatives targeted at music, reminiscence and wellbeing. These initiatives have to rely on some kind of technology, whether acoustic or electronic musical instruments, radios or CD players, iPads or online streaming apps/services. Clearly, our sessions at the two Liverpool care centres depended on the use of digital technologies and raised questions about access to such technologies, and the importance of not taking this for granted. Utilizing these technologies commonly involves not only a degree of economic privilege but also a particular set of skills, knowledge and a willingness to engage with new and changing technologies. Factors such as age and gender can also play a part. For audiences aged 60 and over, media and entertainment technologies in domestic homes, such as televisions, computers and music stereo systems, have tended to be a male preserve, a point highlighted in numerous scholarly studies. In his article '"Turn It down!" She Shrieked: Gender, Domestic Space, and High Fidelity, 1948–59', (1996), for example, the popular music scholar Keir Keightley explains how during the 1950s, hi-fi became associated with men and coded as masculine.

For the sessions at the day-care centres, we wanted to access songs via Spotify, a music streaming service, and YouTube, a video streaming service. Prior to our visit we had been informed that online access was available at the centres but on arrival it was immediately clear that there were various technological challenges for us to confront. The first centre we visited had Wi-Fi but the staff did not know the password, while the second centre was not equipped with the Wi-Fi or Internet access we had been promised. Both centres nevertheless had a CD player that was readily used by the staff in their caring roles, while one of them had a television that was never used. For both workshops we had brought with us a portable Wi-Fi dongle to help access music streaming services. Clearly, however, those using the centres on a regular basis did not have this access. If they wanted to play music recordings they were therefore reliant on the small collection of CDs that each centre had available.

Moreover, the workshops raised questions not only about access to music technology at the day-care centres but also beyond these centres, whether by the centres' users or by older audiences more generally. Some of those who participated in the workshops told us about the music they liked to listen to and in doing so referred to live music events they had attended, and radio programmes or vinyl records they had listened to. Only one person referred to CDs and no one mentioned accessing music through digital technology. Most of those we spoke to either did not have Internet at home or they had it but were unable to access it, either because of a lack of knowledge or because of the physical dexterity required. In their work on 'Social Media and Social Class', Simeon Yates and Eleanor Lockley argue that use of digital media (their focus is on social media) depends not simply on being able to afford it, and to cover the cost of digital products and online subscription services. It also depends on having the skills required to use this technology (2018, pp. 1291–1316).

Lack of access to the Internet, and to digital music technologies and streaming services, were not the only barriers to music listening at home for those participating in our workshops. Other music technologies were also difficult to access: the buttons on their CD players were too small for them to see; the radio needed re-tuning but the knobs could not be twisted because of arthritis; turntables had been broken and were difficult to replace. One participant, Rosie, mentioned that she only ever listened to one CD featuring a recording by

Andrea Bocelli. When asked why, she explained that after losing her sight a few years previously, she had been unable to see to change the CD and replace it in the machine with another. Betty, who was in the same group as Rosie, mentioned that she was a Buddy Holly fan and had all of his records. She used to dance to them with her husband but after her record player had broken, she had not been able to get it fixed and the records were now stored in boxes and unused. Consequently, for these and other participants, musical objects such as records or tape cassettes and music listening had shifted from being part of their everyday life and experience to being an occasional interlude provided by a friend, carer or external organization.

Despite the various challenges and limitations of our encounters with these groups, our visits to the two day-care centres highlighted the benefits of music initiatives for remembering and wellbeing. This final part of our chapter focusses on one important benefit, which concerns music's unique role in the forging of social relationships and identities.

CONNECTING TO SELF AND OTHERS THROUGH MUSIC

When we listened back to the recordings of the workshops it became clear that some interesting stories were being told and shared by the participants as they listened to the music. In her article 'Preservation of self in people with dementia living in residential care: A socio-biographical approach' (2006), Claire Surr, a Professor of Dementia Studies, explores how people understand and contextualize *self* through storytelling and self-narration. Drawing on interviews with 14 care home residents who were living with dementia, Surr analyzes the stories they told and the narrative conventions involved. Whether stories of a life or of selected life events, or stories with possible meta-phorical interpretations, Surr explains how they helped her interviewees to maintain a sense of self, and to contextualize and position this self in relation to the past. This maintenance of self was likewise evident in the stories and 'I' statements that were prompted by the music at our care centre sessions: 'I love Buddy Holly', 'Oh, my husband hated Buddy Holly he was an Elvis Fan', 'Me and my sister used to go see all the Elvis films. We loved getting dressed up and going to the pictures.' There are some direct correspondences here with the responses of participants at Lisa's series of workshops at the Memory Film Club in Brazil, where the use of the subject pronoun 'eu' (often an emphatic 'I' in Portuguese) was notable in recounting their reminiscences (see Chapter 3, pp. 129–130).

During our visits to the two day-care centres, we found that by sharing music and listening experiences together, some of those using these centres were able to establish connections with one another: Tom Jones was clearly a favourite, and some of those at the first centre we visited were familiar with the lyrics of songs such as 'Delilah' and 'Green, Green Grass of Home', and able to sing along together. Tammy Wynette's 'Stand by your Man' prompted a similar response, and one of the carers helped by providing us with a countdown to the chorus, while 'Blanket on the Ground' by Billie Jo Spears was accompanied by both singing and handclapping. When Sally suddenly remembered the song 'Naughty Lady on Shady Lane', some of the other group members tried to help her identify the singer so that we could play it. Jacky looked it up online and informed us that it was a Dean Martin song. She played it. Tammy Wynette was next and they all sang along. The other table joined in, with the carer in full voice (she counted us all into the chorus).

Sometimes there were considerable difficulties in estab-lishing connections between the group members. To give one example, Teresa and Mary were sitting next to each other when we tried to engage them in conversation on their musical past and what they remembered about it. Mary was well-groomed, smartly dressed and highly articulate but unable to comment on music from the past, and told us that she could not remember anything. Teresa, who was the same age as Mary but looked a lot older, clearly loved music and was desperate to talk to us about it. Her smile never waned, her eyes gleamed, she swayed and sang along to the music, her head nodded enthusiastically as we spoke, and her responses to our questions were immediate. She nevertheless found it difficult to make herself understood. There were memories and experiences she wanted to share but we struggled to understand what she was saying, and were forced to grab onto the odd word or rely on non-verbal communication. At one point, it became evident that she and her sister used to frequent a club called the Ambrose where they would sing along to music. Mary did not know Teresa and tried to use this club to establish a connection, and some common ground. She thought she remembered going to the Ambrose, she explained, and seeing Teresa there. She asked Teresa about it but could not understand Teresa's replies, so tried to simplify things by asking Teresa who she used to sit with. When Teresa mentioned her sister, Mary asked what her sister's name was and where she was now, so Teresa explained that her sister had died. Over the ensuing minutes Mary asked Teresa the same questions over and over again, which meant that Teresa kept having to repeat that her sister, who she had clearly been close to, was dead.

Despite such difficulties, it was clear from our centre visits that music provided a focus for shared remembering that not only re-established a sense of self, but also a connection to others in the present. Similarly, as the group members listened to the music we played most of them were able to externalize their remembering and share it with the other group members, not only by singing along but also through their gestures and facial expressions. Following the visual media scholar Annette Kuhn, these responses to the music can be described as 'performances of memory'. In her article on film, photography and memory (2010), Kuhn shows how the past can be re-enacted through performances of memory both in and with visual media. She uses this to emphasize the 'doing' of memory and the effort and work involved, something clearly illustrated by the exchanges between Mary and Teresa as they struggled to remember their visits to the Ambrose club, and share their experiences of it.

It was not necessary for those at the two care centres to remember the same musical moment or place for these musical connections to take place. One participant, Lilly, had emigrated from Hong Kong as an adult. She was a passionate fan of Tom Jones and despite speaking very little English, she interacted and sang with the other participants when the song 'Green, Green Grass of Home' was played. This moment also highlights how music can connect people across places that are geographically dispersed, while also enabling them to connect with one another in the moment through the live listening experience. The impromptu singalongs were a well-being benefit of the workshops and part of the 'we-ness' of shared experience. People engaged in social interaction regardless of language barriers or starkly contrasting backgrounds, connecting with one another through lived musical experience. Although Sylvia was a regular at the first centre we visited, she was reluctant to join in the singing and stayed at the back of the room. It was only towards the end of the session, when we were about to pack up our equipment in time for lunch, that Sylvia told us about her experiences of music in her home country of Italy. She had been moved to a table in the middle of the room where lunch would be served and mentioned 'That's Amore', performed by Dean Martin. When we played it she immediately burst into song. Swaying along to the music, hands clasped together, she sang at the top of her voice, which encouraged those around her to watch or join in. When we told her how wonderful her voice was she explained that in the part of Italy where she and her family lived, the whole community used to gather outside to sing: 'the older and the younger would all join in, but they don't do that now'.

Moments like these illustrate the benefits of listening with others rather than through headphones. Headphone listening is, by its very nature, an individualistic experience because only the person wearing the headphones is able to hear the music. Although this has some benefits, it does not allow for the social benefits of collective listening and musical moments that can be shared. The ability to talk and respond to the music as soon as it was played was important, and conversations would often start while a song was playing. Participants shared a collective experience of music as well as being able to share stories together, with carers and family members in some cases. While *Playlist for Life* advocates headphone listening, it can be an isolating experience when only one person can listen at a time. It can also be problematic in terms of resourcing if multiple MP3 players and headphones are required, as might be the case with listening in care centres. More importantly, perhaps, for older people like those at the care centres we visited, headphone listening has never been a normalized part of their listening experience. While the approach taken by *Playlist for Life* involves listening to music that speaks to an individual's personal history, limiting this to headphone listening diminishes the way this music can enhance social interaction, storytelling, reminiscence and, by extension, the sense of 'we-ness' and wellbeing benefits of the activity. The shared experience of music, whether listening to a record together, participating with others in a live performance or singing together, is important. It helps, for example, to tackle isolation and connect people to others, and to maximize the wellbeing potential of music-centred interventions and initiatives.

CONCLUSION

The increasing popularity of music as a tool for improving wellbeing has led to a proliferation of related programmes, workshops and interventions. Run by charities and various cultural organizations and businesses, this chapter has described initiatives that highlight particular ways in which music can support remembering and 'healthy ageing'. It is nevertheless not always clear what the purpose or rationale of a particular initiative is and whether, for example, the aim is to prompt remembering by stimulating activity in the brain (as seen in the film documentary *Alive Inside*) or physical activity (as with the charity *Singing for Brain* whose activities are designed to prompt both memory and physicality). There is nevertheless clear evidence from a range of organizations that involvement in singing and other music-making activities can benefit older audiences, and those living with dementia and age-related memory loss. What we have argued in this chapter is that listening to recorded music can bring similar benefits. Listening is not necessarily a passive experience but an activity that everyone can engage with and participate in. It can therefore bring people together and enable a shared experience. Moreover, as we learned from our visits to day-care centres in Liverpool, through this listening individuals can connect with others in the present, while also connecting with a self that existed in the past.

Bringing people together to listen collectively can be facilitated in many different ways; these shared listenings can encourage reminiscence, connectivity and 'we-ness' amongst participants, carers and families. We have a few 'best-practice' suggestions that are useful if you want to run a 'Music and Wellbeing' session:

- First of all, try to find a space where there are no noisy distractions so that people can focus on the music.

- Start the music, whether it is the radio or a CD, a tape, a live performance or an old record. Music may spark stories from the past or connect people in the present, and making time to listen together can support 'we-ness' and connectiveness between people.

- Let the music produce an effect; not every song sparks a memory or moves you to tears but sometimes a song comes on that you just cannot help but sing along to. There are also songs that make us dance or cry, that move us to remember a moment from the past. It is important to support people in these moments; this might mean holding their hand or dancing along with them but it is important that we can be with people in that moment and share a glimpse of the memories that the particular track holds.

- Give space to talk, since we cannot always predict what music will resonate with someone. For example, we would never have predicted Lilly's love of Tom Jones or Rosie living with the soundtrack of Andrea Bocelli. We would not have learned the importance of these songs if we had not created space for people to share their listening experiences. We can often be tempted to just let music run from track to track, but taking time to share reactions to music together and talk about people's preferences can help us to understand one another better.

3

MUSIC AND FILM IN DEMENTIA CARE IN BRAZIL AND ON MERSEYSIDE

Lisa Shaw and Clarissa Giebel

Dementia care need not be a relatively passive attendance upon an elderly man or woman's psychological undoing. Rather, it may become an exemplary model of interpersonal life, an epitome of how to be human.

–Kitwood and Bredin (1992, p. 286).

DEMENTIA, PERSONHOOD AND WELLBEING

Hampson and Morris (2016) argue that the way we view a person with dementia can have a significant effect on their level of disability and wellbeing. Accepting that the cognitive dysfunction stemming from dementia disrupts a person's sense of being in the world or sense of self, they support the view that rather than disintegrating, leaving a non-person, the self remains in those living with dementia, and although mis-placed, this self can be maintained with appropriate care

(Hampson & Morris, 2016, pp. 1–6). It is widely accepted that in order to increase the wellbeing of people with dementia it is essential to foster and preserve their sense of self, what is often referred to as their 'personhood', the way someone relates to others socially. Engagement with other people – what academics refer to as 'intersubjectivity' – is therefore key to good dementia care. Kitwood and Bredin have persuasively shown how people with dementia can display varying degrees of 'wellbeing' or conversely 'ill-being' in a way that does not map directly on to their level of cognitive impairment (1992, p. 275):

> *Some who have long since reached around zero score on all cognitive tests still appear to be faring well as persons. Others whose cognitive powers are only moderately impaired appear to be faring far less well. A dementing condition tends to be compounded by depression or anxiety, a sense of apathy or disencouragement. It makes good sense, then, to speak of a dementia sufferer as being in a state of relative well-being or ill-being, in a way that cuts across the dimension of cognitive impairment.*
> (Kitwood & Bredin, 1992, p. 280)

These academics understand a definition of wellbeing as being contingent on a sense of personhood and hinging on four key characteristics of a person with dementia (all of which are highly dependent on the quality of care they receive), as follows: personal worth or self-esteem; a sense of agency and ability to control one's personal life in a meaningful way; social confidence, the feeling of being at ease with others and having something to offer them; and hope, the retention of confidence or trust that some security will remain. Kitwood and Bredin continue:

> *It is often the case that a dementia sufferer who is*
> *visibly withdrawing, or becoming demoralized, is*
> *transformed by a little real attention and human*
> *contact. It is as if he or she needs to be re-called to the*
> *world of persons, where a place is no longer*
> *guaranteed. At such times one or more of the*
> *indicators of wellbeing may be shown, only to fade*
> *quickly. Wellbeing, then, for dementia sufferers,*
> *often appears to be fragile and short-lived. Whereas*
> *some individuals with the full range of cognitive*
> *powers have inner reserves to draw on, or at least*
> *well-developed capacities for carrying on in a 'frozen'*
> *state, those who are some way into a dementing*
> *illness do not. Often they seem to have virtually no*
> *reserves, and to be drifting towards the threshold of*
> *unbeing. Their personhood needs to be continually*
> *replenished, their selfhood continually evoked and*
> *reassured.* (1992, p. 285)

By focussing on the perspective of personhood in dementia care, and moving away from the biomedical model, it has been argued that the symptoms/behaviour and the quality of life of a person with dementia are the result of that person's social interactions with others rather than of neurological changes (O'Connor et al., 2007). Some aspects of these research conclusions have been particularly useful when formulating our projects and the toolkit; via group reminiscence and personal interaction in small groups or even one to one, we have sought to reassure participants living with dementia that they are individuals with a past and a continued identity who have stories that we are interested in and thus 'have something to offer'. We have also tried to involve these people in shaping the projects, eliciting ideas from them and encouraging them to take part in related activities, such as making props and costumes. Our ethos is that even if 'fragile and short-lived', the wellbeing benefit of increasing their sense of agency in this way, of boosting their social confidence and sense of ease among other people, is still worthwhile.

We have aimed to extend the duration of this sense of wellbeing by encouraging users of the toolkit to embed their film-related reminiscence sessions into a wider programme of related activities that becomes part of the routine of the participants, over a period of several weeks or months, if not more permanently. As Chaudhury (1999, p. 232) has stated: 'For people with dementia, memory for recent life experiences may be impaired more than memories of distant times, places, and events', so the use of film material that dated from the adolescence and early adulthood of the participants (the 'memory' or 'reminiscence bump') seemed particularly appropriate for use with people living with a dementia diagnosis.[1] We were inspired, in part, by the BBC Reminiscence Archive, first established in 2016, which provides access to a selection of content from the BBC Archives – including photos, videos and sound clips – that is designed to support reminiscence therapy. This material is organized by theme or decade, and search results are randomized on each visit to the website, although they can be 'favourited' to return later.[2] This material could easily be used by carers and occupational therapists, drawing on the techniques outlined in our toolkit, as part of longer-term *Cinema, Memory and Wellbeing* therapeutic interventions. The sense of personhood, while unarguably enhanced by the various personalized tools we

---

1 For further discussion, see the definition in the Introduction (p. 26), Chapter 2 (pp. 90–91) and the article by Rathbone, Moulin, and Conway (2008).

2 See, for example, the BBC's archive collection of television shows from the 1950s such as *The Generation Game*. https://remarc.bbcrewind.co.uk/content.html?content=video&theme=TV%20and%20Radio.

discussed in the Introduction, such as a personal digital memory bank using the *House of Memories* app, a *Playlist for Life* and various other stimuli, has been shown to be drawn out most effectively in group situations, where people are encouraged to perform their sense of self to others. Group reminiscence therapy has been shown to be promising for improving wellbeing and reducing depressive symptoms among institutionalized older adults (Gaggioli et al., 2014), and for those living with a dementia diagnosis group reminiscence therapy can help foster an emotional connection between group members, as well as reducing anxiety by providing focus and distraction, as the questionnaire responses to our first workshops discussed in Chapter 1 suggest. By discussing topics from the past that they are all familiar with, group members form a common ground and sense of belonging.[3] Through these shared memories, a fragile sense of self can be reaffirmed and new friendships established, tackling issues of isolation and loneliness which can be felt by group members even in a crowded room. For these reasons our approach in all the projects we discuss in this book has been to work with groups of people rather than individuals on a one-to-one basis.

USING THE TOOLKIT WITH BRAZILIANS LIVING WITH DEMENTIA

The toolkit (available in English and in Portuguese) has evolved in key stages as the various pilot projects have developed. The first step was making contact with a local

---

3 The Disabled Living Foundation's factsheet 'Living with Dementia: leisure and reminiscence activities' https://www.dlf.org.uk/factsheets/leisure-reminiscence-activities#5.

nursing home, asking its staff to suggest how they could best be supported and then working with experienced professionals at the University of Liverpool in designing the tools for measuring wellbeing, as discussed in Chapter 1. The following stage was to move up to the next level of care provision by working city-wide with a local council in Brazil, with an NHS health trust in the UK and with the management team of large private care providers in both countries. As Clarissa has explored in her research, there has been a growing interest internationally in how non-pharmacological interventions can help people living with a dementia diagnosis continue to live in their own homes and assist them in maintaining everyday functional independence for as long as possible. Clarissa has also highlighted, however, that when developing such interventions, country-specific variations should be considered, including such factors as whether the local culture deems that older people should be cared for in the home by family members for their entire lives, and whether there is any national policy on dementia (the latter not always existent even in Europe) (Giebel et al., 2014). The lack of a national policy on dementia in Brazil is reflected in the dramatic underdiagnosis of the disease and the absence of a culture of dementia care. As Engedal and Laks conclude:

> *In Brazil, where an estimated 1.6 million people have dementia, only around one in four has been assessed and diagnosed. A nationwide dementia plan could both increase the number of people being diagnosed, but above all would improve the quality of care and quality of life for people with dementia and their families. Brazil can learn from the European plans which success factors and barriers are of importance, and how to implement new and better services for people with dementia.* (2016, p. 78)

We were therefore keen to expand the Brazilian pilot project and encourage use of the Portuguese-language version of the toolkit to embrace older people living with a dementia diagnosis. Well aware of the considerable challenges of doing so, given the national context, Lisa sought the help of the local city council in Petrópolis, where the pilot project had been conducted. She asked her contacts at the Fazenda Inglesa GP practice, notably the GP and the practice nurse, to put her in touch with key contacts in the council. She wanted to identify local nursing homes that specialized in dementia care, and to find an enthusiastic partner institution to work with. After being introduced face to face to Gabriela de Almeida Falconi, President of the Petrópolis CMDDPI (Municipal Board for the Defence of the Rights of Older People) at a council meeting that was open to the public, Lisa was invited by Gabriela to present the project and its proposed expansion to a meeting of the city council in April 2017. She subsequently received a letter of recommendation from the CMDDPI, recognizing the project as an example of best practice and encouraging its adoption more broadly in the city.[4] Lisa was then invited to hold a *Cinema, Memory and Wellbeing* session for older people on 5 October 2017 at the Terra Santa Educational Centre in Petrópolis, as part of the commemorations of UNESCO's International Day of Older Persons. The audience was made up of some 60 residents and users of a range of care facilities and nursing homes in the city, some of whom had received a dementia diagnosis, and was covered in the local press. A representative from Petrópolis city council summarized the positive outcomes as follows:

---

4 See http://www.petropolis.rj.gov.br/pmp/index.php/imprensa/noticias/item/ 7333-semana-do-idoso-promove-atividade-em-parceria-com-universidade- de-liverpool.html.

> *The participants interacted throughout the event,*
> *remembering their youth. Many said they*
> *remembered the films shown in the event. Those*
> *present at the event went on a happy journey back in*
> *time and experienced the joy of being able to re-live*
> *those memories. My evaluation is that all the older*
> *people enjoyed the event. Some of them were shy*
> *when they arrived but as the event went on, they*
> *opened up and talked to each other, telling their*
> *stories and sharing their experiences with those*
> *present out loud. I believe the presentation was*
> *productive and suggested that we do more of them as*
> *soon as possible.*

A representative of the Terra Santa Educational Centre, which kindly offered to host the event free of charge, gave the following equally positive feedback:

> *They [the older attendees] had the opportunity to*
> *recapture the past by remembering their childhood*
> *and youth. They were happy to be able to share*
> *moments of their lives. It was of great value to the*
> *third age since they found the old films nostalgic, and*
> *they were thus able to recapture memories from their*
> *past that were important.*

As an intermediary to the city council with extensive knowledge of and contacts with the care home sector in the city of Petrópolis and the surrounding area, Gabriela Falconi subsequently set up a meeting between Lisa and the then manager of the Lar São João de Deus nursing home in the outlying district of Itaipava, a centre of excellence for dementia care. The mission statement of this nursing home at the time included the aim of becoming, by 2019, the best long-stay home for older people in the mountain region of the state of Rio de Janeiro, and its management saw the benefits of training its staff to use the *Cinema, Memory and Wellbeing* toolkit to enhance provision for its residents, particularly those living with a dementia diagnosis. They especially liked the toolkit's emphasis on group interaction and community wellbeing, and its use of Brazilian musical comedy films that would resonate with its residents. According to its resident psychologist: 'This type of humanized intervention for older people promotes the holistic vision of our organization. Our greatest aim is to ensure that this is in fact a Home, a place of safety, joy, comfort and affection.' The management of this private-sector home was also keen to highlight this innovative wellbeing activity in its marketing material. The partnership thus proved relatively easy to establish – the key, in Lisa's experience, is to find a partner institution – and one or more individuals within – that are enthusiastic about the project and then to listen carefully to their particular needs and adapt the project accordingly. After an initial planning meeting, and detailed email exchanges outlining the proposed project and adapting the methodology of the toolkit to fit the needs and established routine of the nursing home in question, Lisa ran a four-week 'Memory Film Club' between July and August 2018, where participants included those living with a diagnosis of dementia-related mild cognitive impairment.

THE LAR SÃO JOÃO DE DEUS NURSING HOME'S 'MEMORY FILM CLUB'

Participants in the 'Memory Film Club' included residents of the nursing home (some with dementia-related mild cognitive impairment) and members of the local community who

attended the Father Fernandes Activity Centre, a day facility
that allows non-residents to benefit from activities run by the
nursing home free of charge. The majority were aged over 65
years, although a couple of younger non-residents also
attended to accompany older friends or relatives. The participants were selected by the care home's psychologist, in
consultation with its Executive Director and GP/gerontologist,
the residents/day users themselves and their family members.
All participants were able to give informed consent to
participate in the project, in line with the ethical requirements
of the University of Liverpool's Ethics Committee.

Once a week, for four weeks, in groups of about 20 people
(combining a mix of residents and non-residents, living with
and without a dementia diagnosis) participants watched a
different audio-visual presentation made up of carefully
selected short clips from Brazilian musical comedies from the
1950s, such as so-called *chanchada* films made by the Atlân-
tida and Cinedistri studios. These were films that participants
were likely to have seen in their teenage years/early adulthood
and thus aimed to draw on the 'reminiscence' or 'memory
bump' identified by academics, as noted earlier. Immediately
after each clip, Lisa, as well as the home's psychologist, care
assistants (*agentes de ação social*), and the newly arrived
resident priest, interacted with the group, asking open questions about any possible memories that had come to mind and
chatting to the participants, paying attention and giving
importance to their responses. Different types of clips were
chosen, based on Lisa's research into the films of this era
(Bergfelder et al., 2017; Dennison & Shaw, 2004; Shaw &
Dennison, 2007), as follows: those containing famous Brazilian film stars, such as Oscarito, Grande Otelo, Nancy
Wanderley and Zezé Macedo, who collectively represented
different ethnic and regional backgrounds, thus increasing the
chances of audience identification – particularly with popular

stars as we mentioned in the Introduction (Stacey, 1993); music and dance numbers featuring well-known performers like Eliana Macedo, Emilinha Borba and Ivon Curi; and sequences featuring recognizable locations such as the nearby Hotel Quitandinha in Petrópolis and the iconic Copacabana Palace hotel in the city of Rio de Janeiro. Each presentation lasted around 45 minutes and was paused after every 5- to 10-minute clip. This short-clip format (rather than the screening of entire feature-length films) aimed to maintain the attention of all participants, allow for 'comfort breaks' as necessary and optimize the reminiscence potential of film material by creating what Annette Kuhn (2010) calls a 'memory text', wherein the lack of a coherent linear narrative provides 'non-identificatory points of entry for the viewer, spaces inside which her or his own memories and processes of remembering may be activated' and subsequently shared with the rest of the group in a process of collective, shared remembering (Kuhn, 2010, p. 299). The choice of a mixture of types of clips was also inspired by recent studies into the relationship between wellbeing among older people and music and humour, respectively (for example, Houston et al., 1998; MacDonald, Kreutz, & Mitchell, 2012; Tse et al., 2010), and allowed for evaluation of the relative effectiveness of music/ song, humour and star/location recognition in generating reminiscence.

When applying for funding – in Lisa's case for research projects, but equally for resources to put on additional events in the case of activities coordinators in care homes or occu-pational therapists – the need to provide 'evidence' of well-being benefits cannot be avoided. To capture this evidence, the project used a similar mixed-methods methodology to that piloted at the nursing home in Liverpool, including quantita-tive and qualitative methods to generate data and measure wellbeing benefits of the 'Memory Film Club'. The aim was to capture and measure any improvements in positive mood, self-esteem, confidence and sociability, and any reduction in anxiety, negative mood and social isolation. It was also intended that the group interaction itself would generate an added wellbeing benefit and contribute to the cognitive process. However, as had been the case in the pilot project on Merseyside, measuring these potential benefits in a systematic way proved to be difficult and counter-productive from a wellbeing perspective. In week one, Lisa used a brief questionnaire based on the 'Measures Umbrellas and Generic Wellbeing scale' developed by University College London (UCL Museum Wellbeing Measures Toolkit), to see if it would be more user-friendly and would generate more systematic results than the questionnaires used in the pilot study at the nursing home in Liverpool.[5] This material was translated into Portuguese and the intention was for Lisa and the resident psychologist to pose the questions orally in individual sessions with the participants immediately before and after each weekly film presentation. In practice, this method was only adopted in week one because it proved both time-consuming and too complicated for the participants. It clearly destroyed the anticipation of the cinema session, with one participant complaining that she was bored now and wanted to leave the room before the screening had even commenced. Lisa therefore adapted the measurement tool for week two, asking participants to choose from a list of adjectives to describe their mood before and after the film activity. This proved to engage them more, although they still tended to opt for 'well' at the beginning and 'well' or 'very well' at the end, a similar problem to the one we had experienced at the nursing home in

---

5 The Measures Umbrella and Generic Wellbeing questionnaire can be downloaded at https://www.ucl.ac.uk/culture/sites/culture/files/ucl_museum_wellbeing_measures_toolkit_sept2013.pdf.

relation to a question about happiness, as we discussed in Chapter 1. In weeks three and four, Lisa chose a different approach – the lesson is to be prepared for things not to work out as planned and be ready to try out different methods until you find one that works best. Lisa wanted to obtain more detailed feedback from the audience on how the sessions left them feeling, so she engaged the help of the psychologist, the care assistants and the resident priest, and they each sat with individual participants at the end of the session and simply asked how he or she was feeling. Some of the responses are reproduced below, and in our view provide ample evidence of the immediate wellbeing benefits of the activity:

Participant 1: 'I loved it. After [the 'Memory Film Club' sessions] I feel really good. It was just what we needed. It brings back good memories. We re-live those times'.

Participant 2: 'I feel uplifted afterwards, as light as a feather. It's always good to remember our childhood'.

Participant 3: '[I feel] good. I've left my problems out there. Here [in the 'Memory Film Club'] there's just joy'.

Participant 4: '[I feel] more relaxed, it took my mind off things – it made me forget my worries. Good times!'

Participant 5: '[I feel] good. Very good. I leave here very cheerful'.

In Lisa's view, posing open questions on a one-to-one basis elicits much more convincing 'evidence' of the wellbeing benefits of this activity, and this is powerfully complemented by the physical reactions of the participants (laughter, chatter, smiles, breaking into song, moving to the music and so on), and particularly the animated interaction that spontaneously occurred in the breaks between the clips and at the end of the session, all of which were recorded on audio and are described in more detail below. One-to-one discussions with people living with dementia have the added value of showing that person that they still have something to contribute – an essential aspect of wellbeing, as noted above – and that someone is interested in what they have to say. (Many of the participants in the 'Memory Film Club', including those with a dementia diagnosis, made a point of commenting on how important and even surprising it was to them that someone found their memories of interest.) Lisa and the resident psychologist also used the participant observation technique, taking notes during the periods of audience interaction, and thus collecting data in the least obtrusive way possible and not distracting the participants or hindering their enjoyment.

To add weight to the research dimension of the 'Memory Film Club', Lisa conducted semi-structured individual interviews with the nursing home staff directly involved (psychologist and care assistants [*agentes de ação social*], and the resident priest) in week one and week four of the project, all of which were recorded on audio for subsequent transcription and analysis. The staff all gave examples of participants whose behaviour had changed in a positive way in the course of the project. The priest observed that one of the male participants in particular had surprised him. This man has considerable speech difficulties, but immediately after one of the sessions he asked the priest if he could do some readings during mass. The priest firmly believes that this change in behaviour was due to the fact that this man had gained self-confidence as the project went on, speaking about his personal reminiscences more in each session. One of the care assistants made the following statement: 'I have discovered how to work with them [the older people] through this project. So, I can build on the project from now on. Let them talk more […] and listen, give them more attention. Awaken their curiosity.' The priest summarized the benefits of the project as follows:

> *It gives value to their [the older people's] lives as they are. They are people with a history. They can feel that today, for us, the history they have lived through in the past continues to be important. That has made a big difference to them. It has been very useful for me, enabling me to create closer links with them.*

After the final session of the film club in week four, the nursing home hosted a grand finale party, which all the participants attended wearing simple costume jewellery and headdresses inspired by Carmen Miranda that they had created themselves during weekly arts and crafts workshops held over the previous four weeks and led by the resident psychologist. They had also made decorations for the party venue, and a gift for Lisa of a photograph album made from old vinyl records (which included photos of participants taken throughout the previous weeks). The party was a great success, and Lisa used it as an opportunity to thank all the participants and the staff by presenting each of them with a souvenir – a mug that they could use every day during the tea and coffee breaks that was decorated with photographs taken during the 'Memory Film Club' sessions. Themed souvenirs were also given to the participants in our project on Merseyside with Company Matters4U – coasters that doubled as small jigsaws to improve dexterity – and to the Brazilian participants in the pilot project at the Fazenda Inglesa GP practice – fridge magnets featuring images of local film stars from the 1950s and the details of the film event. This is a simple way of creating a talking point for carers and visitors and reminding the participants of the event in the days, weeks and months that follow, thus maximizing its potential well-being benefits.

MAINTAINING PERSONHOOD WHEN LIVING
WITH DEMENTIA

*In terms of the metaphor of states of personhood, the
self that is shattered in dementia will not naturally
coalesce; the Other [person] is needed to hold the
fragments together. As subjectivity breaks apart, so
intersubjectivity must take over if personhood is to be
maintained. At a psychological level, this may be
understood as the true agenda for dementia care.*
–Kitwood and Bredin (1992, p. 285).

In this section we will look at some concrete examples of
how a variety of short film clips, some of which include music,
can be used in a group setting to help people with a dementia
diagnosis relate to others and thereby perform a sense of self
through communicating, what the academics cited above refer
to as 'intersubjectivity' and a crucial way of establishing
'personhood' and thus stimulating wellbeing as we discussed
in the Introduction. The first example relates to the second
week of the 'Memory Film Club' at the Lar São João de Deus
nursing home in Brazil, and explores the responses of a group
of residents with early-stage dementia. During the screening of
clips from the musical comedy *É de chuá!* (It's Fab!, Victor
Lima, 1958), when they heard the song "Madureira chorou"
("Madureira cried"), one of the major hits of the Rio de
Janeiro carnival in 1958, many members of the group began
to smile, move to the music and sing along. A number of them
immediately burst into song, joining in the easily remembered
chorus. Although they did not know all the words, they
hummed to the music, some of them moving to the rhythm as
they sat in their chairs, and most joined in whenever the
refrain was repeated. When the clip ended, they began to chat
animatedly with their neighbours and the chatter did not die

down for several minutes. One woman did not recognize the singer performing the song in the film clip (Joel de Almeida) but sang a few lines from the song and said "I think it's Gilberto Alves" (she was not correct but that did not matter to her – the song was much more significant than the artist). The same woman then began talking about Madureira, a neighbourhood of Rio de Janeiro referenced in the song's lyrics and title: "Madureira was the focus of...[hesitation] ... samba, samba was there in Madureira". The group then started talking about carnival, the carnival social clubs or so-called 'samba schools' (escolas de samba) and their rehearsals. Improvising, Lisa then posed a series of questions adapted to fit around their spontaneous comments:

Lisa: 'Does this song bring back any specific memory or any memory of carnival in the old days?'

Woman A: 'My parents! They loved this. My father loved this. He worked, arrived at home at five in the afternoon, got his record player, turned it on in the living room, would turn the horn that way ... He was mad about it, sitting us all there to listen'

Woman B: 'Carnival in the Post Office Square. It was street carnival. It was a wonderful'.

Woman C: 'I first danced in carnival aged six. I was a child'.

Woman D: 'I took part in carnival a lot. I loved it!'

Lisa: 'Do you remember any carnival costume you wore?'

Woman A: 'My dad wouldn't let me [dress up]'.

Woman D: 'No, not fancy dress. I had several friends. We used to wear the same clothes. A cute little full skirt, a blouse, or shorts, Bermuda shorts... We were a little group, some ten, twelve people. We all wore the same clothes just to go the [carnival] club. …. in Nova Iguaçú. Sport Clube Nova Iguaçú'. [a working-class suburb of Rio]

Woman B: 'I once wore a *baiana* [Bahian girl] costume to parade where I live … in the carnival *bloco* (street group) … Here. Here in… Pedro do Rio … I never went to carnival in Rio'.

Woman C: 'My costume was a chicken … a bird. I took its head off ….' [she laughed]

Woman D began talking about her childhood in Nova Iguaçú: 'Then they used to put up a stage, put on music… for people to dance to. Those of us who had no money to go to (carnival) club danced there in the street, partying in the street. Like a carnival *bloco* (street group). *Batuquinho* (playing percussion). That thingy. I don't remember the name'. [Lisa prompted: 'Rattle?'] 'That's it!'

In this particular case, a song proved to be a powerful trigger for reminiscence. 'Madureira Chorou' was a well-known carnival song, it became clear, although no one could identify the performer on screen or knew the name of the composers. Its catchy refrain and melody had clearly cemented the song in people's memories, and traditional carnival marches are repeatedly performed in street carnivals on an annual basis, ensuring that old classics like this still feature in the repertoire of even the youngest revellers. The ages of the members of this audience varied between 65 and 93 years, in other words in 1958 they would have ranged in age between 5 and 33 years. Some of them would have taken part in street carnival and listened to the radio, and thus been exposed repeatedly to 'Madureira Chorou', which won the official prize for best carnival samba that year. It evidently also won the popular vote, as various newspaper articles from the time illustrate, with Rio's street carnival groups or *blocos* featuring it prominently in their repertoire, and newspapers publishing its lyrics widely during the carnival period of 1958. The power of the music in this case far outstripped that of the image on screen. During the previous project in Brazil at the Fazenda Inglesa GP practice, a man in his late 70s who had lost his sight a few years earlier and had initially been reluctant to take part in the film session for this reason began to beat a rhythmic accompaniment on his knee on hearing this song. He was visibly moved when he heard it, which initially caused Lisa concern, but he soon reassured her that it had been a very positive experience. 'I travelled through time', he said. 'It took me back to the carnival of my youth in Rio'.

To return to week two's session at the 'Memory Film Club' at the Lar São João de Deus nursing home, the next clip that Lisa showed was from the same musical film (*É de chuá!*) and featured the female star Renata Fronzi wearing a figure-hugging dress, with a narrow waist. No one could remember her name but when Lisa told them it many recalled her and smiled. The images of Fronzi dancing on screen, wearing a tight-fitting satin dress with a nipped-in waist, prompted several women in the audience to interject on the subject of her clothes, and strikingly they related this to themselves, vividly recalling their own outfits from the distant past.

Woman B: 'As well as the tight waist, I had a very full underskirt underneath' [she laughed]

Woman C: 'I had a full skirt that I made myself by hand. […] a full skirt with a tight waist, starched with corn starch. I used to look lovely in it. […] [The dress] had a high neckline, my husband wouldn't let me show any cleavage ... or do my hair, or eyebrows, but I looked beautiful, wonderful'.

Woman B: 'But let me add something. Our knickers weren't like they are today. They were like trousers, with elastic here, with a lace trim'. [several women laughed]

Woman C: 'Our bras were made from floor cloths. We wore bras. I made mine by hand. If I didn't I'd have been scolded' [she laughed]

Two women then launched into detailed descriptions of their wedding dresses, with one of them offering to bring in a photograph of her wedding day. Another then recalled what she described as her 'favourite dress': 'it was made from cheap cotton. We were poor [she laughed]. We made our dresses ourselves. Or local seamstresses did. My nickname was Ângela Maria' [the name of a famous Brazilian singer who starred in films in the 1950s].

These reactions struck a chord with Lisa, as she has often noticed how her own mother, herself living with early-stage dementia, animatedly tells her in surprising detail about the lovely clothes she had when she was young, describing vividly the fabric and colour, and how she acquired them (often hand-me-downs or homemade garments, sometimes even inspired by those worn by movie stars). For women of this generation with mild dementia-related cognitive dysfunction, a sense of self or 'personhood' appears to be powerfully asserted through recollections of specific clothes, in the Brazilian case not necessarily glamorous outfits but also carnival costumes, and such memories boost their self-esteem ('I used to look lovely in it'; 'I looked beautiful, wonderful'). In this setting, these women could also assert their personhood by connecting with others in the group; the resident psychologist commented afterwards on how new friendships were clearly being formed as a result of this activity, even between residents who had never or barely spoken to each other before. The female residents with dementia had clearly found a point of connection via these clothes-centred interactions, but equally as important was how the care workers confessed to Lisa later that hearing these women share recollections of their youthful glamour and detailed memories of specific clothes had enabled them to connect with them on a more meaningful level as 'real people' with 'real histories'.

When listening to the recordings of the group interactions stimulated by the 'Memory Film Club' over its four-week run, what struck Lisa about the spontaneous comments made by both the men and women was the way in which they tended to begin each interjection with an assertive 'I'. Even when Lisa posed open questions to the group as a whole that did not specifically elicit a personal response, the audience members, including those living with a dementia diagnosis, generally responded by talking directly about themselves and using the 'I' pronoun emphatically at the beginning of their interjections, and at regular intervals throughout them. In the Portuguese language, the pronoun for 'I' is 'eu', but, as in Spanish, verb endings often make it clear that individuals are referring to themselves, so the 'eu' is often omitted. In fact, it tends only to be used to avoid ambiguity (and therefore in speech used infrequently, as the speaker is clearly the 'I' unless otherwise stated), or to add emphasis. (So 'eu' would be included in a sentence such as 'You don't like my new dress, but I love it!') In the responses given by those living with dementia who took part in the 'Memory Film Club' there is a surprisingly high occurrence of the subject pronoun 'eu'. These results have marked similarities to the ways in which participants in the music workshops, discussed in

Chapter 2, framed their memories: 'I am a Buddy Holly fan'; 'I am a mother'. In this way the respondents brought the recollection directly back to the self, and we would argue, demonstrated how this kind of group of reminiscence, around a stimulus or theme that generates interaction and connection, encourages a sense of personhood. These results, corresponding with many of the responses at the music workshops, feature what we can call specifically 'I statements'. These 'I statements' clearly support the conclusions of experts such as Surr (2006), who has shown how people with dementia understand and contextualize themselves as people or 'selves' through storytelling and/or self-narration. The recollections of this group of people in Brazil can be categorized as a kind of storytelling that is used to maintain a sense of self, one which Surr terms 'the storied reconstruction of elected biographical life events and experience' (2006, pp. 1721–1722).

When audience members with dementia recognized a famous face or a location on screen they tended to smile, and their eyes often lit up, regardless of whether they could put a correct name to the face or place. When Lisa told them the name of the person in question, members of the group often cheered. Connecting with something on screen – whether a sonic element like a song, or a visual element like a movie star or a singer – clearly triggered a positive response, a sense of wellbeing 'in the moment'. We would argue, as we maintained in the Introduction, that whether the memory of this connection or recognition lasted or not is immaterial. Recognition of locations in film clips also led to spontaneous interjections among those with dementia who took part in the 'Memory Film Club' in Brazil, which often centred again on narratives of the self. A clip from the musical comedy *Um Candango na Belacap* (Roberto Farias, 1961) that featured Santos Dumont airport in the city of Rio de Janeiro led one woman to exclaim 'Oh, great. I'm going back in time!' and another to tell the group how she used to take her children there to look at the planes. Other location shots of central Rio in this film led one previously very withdrawn woman to suddenly talk animatedly to her neighbour for over four minutes about how she worked in Rio as a maid when she was young, living with a family near Copacabana beach. She recalled good memories, like the local Roxy cinema and the Confeitaria Colombo tea rooms, but also negative experiences, such as eventually having to run away from her female employee, 'a horrendous woman', after working in her home for eight months. She then recalled how on her first day working for her she had been sent out to buy bread but had got lost, recounting the episode in great detail. Another woman then interjected, recalling all the different neighbourhoods of Rio where she had worked as a live-in nanny from the age of 15 years. Another clip from the same musical comedy film showed the iconic clock tower of the Mesbla department store in Rio's city centre, which is still there today (though the shop itself no longer exists). A different woman in the audience then recalled: 'It had everything, that shop... Electrical appliances, clothes. I used to spend the day there. I went to Mesbla a lot. It had everything.' In a conceptual study that examines reminiscence interventions centred on past places and selfhood for older people, especially those living with dementia in long-term care facilities, Chaudhury (1999) has concluded that reminiscence about events and aspects associated with significant places from the past can enable a potentially therapeutic process of holding onto one's life experiences, and in turn present opportunities for preserving one's sense of self-identity. He writes:

> *Over time, as the self reflects upon the past lived experience, place experiences are once again*

*internally experienced through the process of
reminiscence. [...] In remembering we are
thrust back, transported into the place we recall.
We can be moved back into this place as much as,
and sometimes more than, into the* time *in
which the remembered event occurred.* (1999,
p. 245)

Recollected emotions around remembered places can
reshape the conception of self in affective terms.

*Feelings associated with places [...] may have a
greater possibility of surfacing in remembering than
relatively 'neutral' experiences. The condition of 'I*
think*, therefore I* am' *as an accepted
conceptualisation of sense of self to one's self and
others may be replaced by the created condition of 'I*
feel*, therefore I* am.' *Evidently, this avenue of
rediscovery of the self holds much potential and
challenge in general, and in particularly for
individuals whose sense of self is withering away.*
(Chaudhury, 1999, p. 248)

He concludes that for those living with a dementia diagnosis who can access memories associated with emotions
more than other kinds of memories, feelings are potentially the
pivotal points of his or her sense of self (Chaudhury, 1999,
p. 248).

We noted in Chapter 1 how important images of places in
times past are in prompting reminiscence and asserting a sense
of self for older people, including those living with mild
cognitive impairment. We will now discuss this in greater
detail, in the context of responses to the archival footage of
Liverpool used by carers and occupational therapists as part
of their piloting of the toolkit.

EMBRACING THOSE LIVING WITH DEMENTIA ON MERSEYSIDE

Keen to establish productive partnerships closer to home, Lisa consulted an academic specialist in dementia care at the University of Liverpool, Dr Clarissa Giebel, who suggested that the focus for measuring benefits should be extended to carers, encompassing both the improvement of their professional skills and their own sense of wellbeing, in addition to that of those they care for. Clarissa also suggested establishing links with occupational therapists to identify their needs in terms of the practicalities of dementia care, and recommended that Lisa complete the Good Clinical Practice on-line course on Working with Adults Lacking Capacity, which proved to be very useful not least by providing detailed guidance on the process of obtaining informed consent if someone lacks capacity.

Lisa and Jacky were able to set up a meeting with Helena Culshaw, an independent occupational therapist and former chair of the Royal College of Occupational Therapists. Helena gave invaluable advice, particularly how the *Cinema, Memory and Wellbeing* toolkit could be embedded by occupational therapists into broader interventions, linking the film clips to arts and crafts activities, wider discussions and writing projects. She provided an invaluable list of local and national contacts, including within Mersey Care NHS Foundation Trust. She also recommended that Lisa and Jacky present the *Cinema, Memory and Wellbeing* toolkit at a North West Region Roadshow organized by the Royal College of Occupational Therapists in May 2019. This generated tremendous interest among the occupational therapists in attendance, all of whom were invited to find out more by listening to a *Cinema, Memory and Wellbeing* webinar given by Lisa as part of *Dementia Action Week* in May 2019. As well as giving practical tips about use of the toolkit, the webinar allowed people to sign up for a free copy of it.

Lisa also held a series of meetings with a senior occupational therapist working in a specialist dementia ward at a hospital that forms part of Mersey Care NHS Foundation Trust, Nicola Vollero-Corry, a contact that she established through the Happy Older People (HOP) network in Liverpool. Nicola provided excellent advice on the particular challenges of holding film-related events on the ward and was keen to be involved in piloting the toolkit with patients living with a dementia diagnosis. Nicola's expertise was a key factor in helping Lisa consider how to deal with negative reactions or even distress on the part of participants, such as that experienced by one lady at the nursing home, discussed in Chapter 1. Nicola recommended that such adverse reactions be minimized by implementing the toolkit as part of a wider occupational therapy programme, ideally involving in-house audio-visual events or trips to local cinemas to see dementia-friendly screenings. She recommended that in other contexts where participants have a dementia diagnosis, care workers and/or volunteers or independent carers who the participants are already familiar with should be in attendance throughout the sessions to reduce any potential distress or confusion, and to deal with any adverse emotional reactions or physical discomfort.

Talking about dementia-friendly screenings led Lisa to establish contact with the Plaza Community Cinema in Crosby, Merseyside, which runs regular monthly screenings of this kind with low-level lighting and reduced-volume sound, as well as serving refreshments free of charge during an interval/comfort break. Once again, finding the right partner was key, and the enthusiasm, creativity and energy of Christine Physick, the Plaza's Arts and Education Director, were instrumental in the development of the 'Cinema,

Memory and Wellbeing Festival' in September–October 2019, an exciting new partnership between the University of Liverpool and this dynamic local community cinema (see Fig. 3.1).

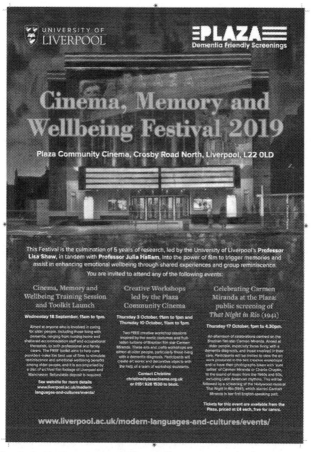

Fig. 3.1. Poster Advertising the Various Events that Composed the *Cinema, Memory and Wellbeing Festival*, a Collaboration between the University of Liverpool and the Plaza Community Cinema, Crosby, Merseyside.

The first event of the 'Festival' was aimed at anyone involved in caring for older people, including those living with dementia, and we publicized it widely via networks of nursing homes, carers (professionals and non-professionals), occupational therapists and sheltered accommodation staff. Thirty-six people attended, and Lisa began the session by asking them to briefly write down on Post-it notes if and how they had already used films in their care of older people or those living with dementia. Lisa then presented the toolkit and an overview of the results of the various projects that had informed it. During a break for refreshments, participants were invited to work in small groups to discuss how they might incorporate any of the ideas that had emerged from Lisa's presentation, and particularly the toolkit itself, to either use film for the first time or to use it differently in their caring roles in future. This led to gratifyingly animated discussions and the formulation of concrete plans (see examples below) about how to embed the toolkit in various contexts. Participants were all given a copy of the toolkit in exchange for agreeing to take part in a follow-up interview some eight weeks later to report back on resulting changes they had implemented.

Some of the plans made by the participants after the presentation of the toolkit demonstrate their understanding of the main points, and how they could incorporate these into existing practices or to embed totally new activities:

- Use short clips rather than whole films, and have pauses for interaction after each (as per our toolkit);

- Ensure the venue has good Internet connection to enable streaming of documentary footage of old Liverpool from the websites listed in the toolkit (as per our toolkit);

- Embed the film screenings in wider projects about local history, perhaps involving local schools and/or online historical archives (as per our toolkit);

- Create playlists of music from the era of the film clips to begin and end the event, and play during the 'interval' while refreshments are served (as we did at the Company Matters4U day-care centres in Liverpool);

- Find different film clips to appeal to different interests, e.g. find content to ensure men are interested and engaged (sports; pubs; working lives etc.) (as per the DVD that accompanies our toolkit);

- Re-enact classic scenes from films as a kind of 'drama' activity, using props and costumes (original idea);

- Put up film posters on the walls (possibly colour photocopies of images from the Internet) and make 'aunt sallies' and rummage boxes containing dressing up clothes etc. (as Lisa did in the Company Matters4U day-care centres and in both projects in Brazil);

- Structure 'film club' into four-week blocks, around a particular theme, and hold related discussion groups (with objects to prompt reminiscence) (as Lisa did in Brazil at the Lar São João de Deus nursing home);

- Integrate film activity into handicrafts project, e.g. to make props (as staff did in Brazil at the Lar São João de Deus nursing home);

- Find out about pots of funding (however small), e.g. to buy a projector; or form partnerships with other institutions to share facilities/participate in each other's events (original idea).

Following this very productive session with carers, the next two events held as part of the *Cinema, Memory and Wellbeing Festival* were two creative workshops, where care home workers and occupational therapists were invited to bring along people with dementia to create Carmen Miranda–inspired props, decorations and headdresses to be worn or displayed at the final screening and celebration. Following the advice of Helena Culshaw to maximize the wellbeing benefits of film screenings in any kind of care setting by integrating them into a wider set of themed activities, we were keen to introduce this new dimension to the project and give participants an active role in preparing decorative objects for the grand finale of the 'Festival', the film screening. This creative component clearly added to the wellbeing benefits of this entire initiative, as evidenced by one of the occupational therapists who attended the first workshop. She commented on how one of her patients with dementia who is habitually disengaged embraced the activity in a surprisingly enthusiastic way, quietly creating a headdress for the entire 90 minutes, and then talking about her granddaughter's interest in fashion design. At the same workshop, another participant with dementia, as she created her headdress, exchanged various recollections that centred on her mother's sewing skills and the lovely clothes she used to make for her as a child and teenager.

The culmination of the 'Festival' was a dementia-friendly screening of the Hollywood musical comedy *That Night in Rio* (Irving Cummings, 1941), starring Carmen Miranda, which all the participants in the workshops and the carers who had attended them, and the initial toolkit training session, were invited to attend. Fancy dress was encouraged, and participants in the workshops wore the articles they had created, as well as sharing spare decorations and props with fellow audience members. The film was screened in the early afternoon, from 1.30 p.m., and was chosen because of its relatively short duration (1 hour and 30 minutes), its eye-catching costumes (shot in Technicolor) and the many song-and-dance numbers that feature in it, including well-known songs that the audience could sing along to. As the spectators arrived, they were welcomed by a local musical duo called *Baiana* performing Carmen Miranda's hit songs and other Brazilian numbers, who also entertained the audience during the 30-minute interval/comfort break, when refreshments were also served. We were very fortunate to come across this local band just a few weeks before the event – and they kindly performed for free, as they share our passion for promoting music as a wellbeing tool. (Similar events could incorporate recorded music instead, choosing CDs that complement the theme and/or era of the film being screened, or perhaps are performed by the musical stars in the film. This was what we had originally planned to do.) We were keen to again provide a souvenir-cum-aide-memoire relating to the event, to derive the greatest possible benefit from it in terms of wellbeing in the short to medium term. We decided to purchase an instant camera and lots of film to enable us to take a photograph of any participant who was interested, either wearing their handmade decorative objects, posing with their heads sticking through an 'aunt sally' of Carmen Miranda or Charlie Chaplin, or just alongside one of us (we were all, by the way, dressed up as Carmen Miranda too!) We obtained written consent to photograph people, from their carers where necessary, when they arrived, or during the interval, while the band were playing. This enabled us to take some of the photographs at the start, some during the interval and the rest at the end of the film screening. This ensured that no one was left out (see Fig. 3.2).

We commissioned a local documentary filmmaker to make a short video about the project, which captures powerful

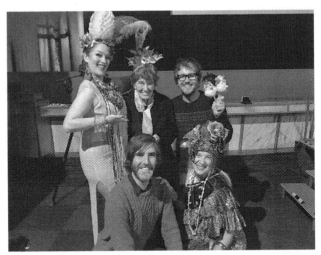

Fig. 3.2. Having Fun after the Screening of the Film *That Night in Rio* at the Plaza Community Cinema, Crosby, Liverpool. Back Row, Left to Right, Laura Doyle (Vocalist of the Group *Baiana* Who Played Live at the Event), Audience Members Lillie Jesse (Wearing a Headdress of Her Own Creation) and Paul Smith; Front Row, Left to Right, Audience Member Stephen Smith and Co-organizer Lisa Shaw.

testimonies from the carers who were involved.[6] One day centre worker commented that her 'service users' seemed to have 'come to life' during the creative workshops, with one lady remembering vividly visiting the same cinema when she was a little girl ('all these memories came flooding back to her and she said it was very touching'). Since the launch of the toolkit and obtaining a copy and the accompanying DVD, this care worker had already used it in the day centre, and she and

---

6 Video of the *Cinema, Memory and Wellbeing Festival* https://vimeo.com/ 368827515/c20a911e12?utm_source=email&utm_medium=vimeo-cliptranscode-201504&utm_campaign=29220.

her colleagues had changed the way they run reminiscence groups, using only shorter clips so people with dementia can retain the information more easily and do not get distracted, and allowing the carers to pause the clips to let them express what they are feeling or want to say. An activities organizer at a local care home said that the wellbeing benefits of the creative workshops clearly lasted for the rest of the afternoon ('it was well past teatime, the staff said the mood lasted, they were full of joy and dancing and singing, so they had a wonderful time, and I'll certainly carry on this scheme. [...] Fantastic initiative. They've had a fabulous time'). By combining a dementia-friendly screening with additional creative activities in a partnership with academics, the Plaza Community Cinema has been inspired to introduce similar events in the future. Its Arts and Education Director, Christine Physick, who had wanted for some time to add a creative dimension to the dementia-friendly screenings she ran but was not sure how to go about it, said: 'it's really made me think about how we could make changes [...] I feel that the partnership enables you to bring a new dimension to your work, sharing and expanding what you are able offer'. The wellbeing benefits in terms of carer resilience were also evidenced in a testimony from another activities coordinator at a specialist dementia care home:

> Working in a home with [people living with] dementia gets overwhelming some days and I was really struggling the last couple of days [...] to get a little lift, and as soon as I saw this [advertised] it lit me up, it gave me hope, and knowing that you do workshops that we can get involved in really helps.

She went on to explain that she has sole responsibility for entertaining 25 residents, and that she struggles to be able to give them all attention in one day. She felt strongly that putting on similar events using film and music in the care home would be extremely helpful, making her job easier and the experience of the residents more fun, as it is difficult to keep the momentum going all day long. She added 'running something like this film festival within the home would be amazing, because all their eyes light up when there's colour and liveliness and music and films, they all enjoy that'.

CONCLUSIONS AND FUTURE DEVELOPMENTS

Lisa Shaw and Julia Hallam

Since we embarked on the first of our projects back in 2014, the subject of dementia and how society needs to give greater importance to finding ways of providing appropriate care and therapeutic interventions has been increasingly in the headlines in the UK and far beyond. Well-known British actress Dame Barbara Windsor, diagnosed with Alzheimer's disease in 2014 and now requiring round-the-clock care, has helped raise the profile of the disease, becoming an ambassador for the Alzheimer's Society and the figurehead of its Fix Dementia Care campaign, which urges the British government to make dementia care a priority and address the crisis in appropriate care provision. As the Alzheimer's Society underlines on its website: 'People affected by dementia typically spend £100,000 on their own care due to a system that is unfair, unsustainable and in need of urgent overhaul. We want to make sure that people with dementia are able to access the care they deserve, when they need it.'[1] Several of Dame

---

1 https://www.alzheimers.org.uk/news/2019-08-28/alzheimers-society-appoints-dame-barbara-windsor-and-husband-scott-mitchell

Barbara's former co-stars in the BBC soap opera *Eastenders* ran the 2019 London marathon as part of the Dementia Revolution campaign, to raise £100,000 to fund dementia research. On the other side of the world, 90-year-old Australian Lorna Prendergast recently completed a Masters in Music and Dementia after being inspired by seeing a television programme on the subject.[2] Her story was shared on social media across the planet. Such headlines have helped to increase awareness of the disease, putting faces and real-life stories to the cold statistics that can often mean very little to us.

As our projects have developed, so have ideas about the benefits of social prescribing. As we noted in the introduction, health-care professionals are becoming increasingly aware of the ways in which a wide range of activities, from Tai Chi and Yoga to dance, singing and creative arts and crafts, can combat isolation and loneliness thereby enhancing wellbeing. In October 2019, the UK government announced plans to create a National Academy for Social Prescribing. The aim is to spread the benefits of non-medical community-based interventions to all, with a particular emphasis on those who suffer from mental health issues, depression and dementia. The Academy aims to train over 1,000 link workers by 2020/ 2021, with over 900,000 people joining a wide range of community schemes.[3] We anticipate that our toolkit can make a small but significant contribution to these ambitions. We have received a growing number of requests from individuals and organizations to provide copies of the *Cinema, Memory*

---

2 https://www.abc.net.au/classic/read-and-watch/music-reads/lorna-prendergast-music-and-dementia/11527196?fbclid=IwAR09s6Ur9I7 kJQ14RZogUnMgbsEBsO5wo922qHJSiCDjmQZ9tzQ-7G2yQy4

3 https://www.gov.uk/government/news/social-prescribing-new-national-academy-set-up

and Wellbeing toolkit and to train people to use it, as well as to give public and more specialist academic lectures about aspects of our projects. These have ranged from people caring for a family member in the home in our local community and in places Lisa has worked in Brazil, to regional groups of occupational therapists who care for people with a range of needs. Given this clear demand for cost-effective solutions that require minimal investment of time (something which is a luxury within the daily routine, as anyone working in the care sector or looking after a loved one will know), we have developed at the University of Liverpool a 'Short Course for Carers: Music, Movies and Memory Tools for Wellbeing in Later Life', to be run by the Department of Continuing Education. This short course is aimed at anyone who is involved in caring for older people, including those living with a dementia diagnosis. It will appeal to professional carers working in nursing homes, day-care centres and independently, occupational therapists, volunteers and those who look after family members. It will run across a six-week period and will explore the basic principles of how music and films can most effectively be used to stimulate memories and reminiscence among older people and those living with dementia; and how to use film- and music-related reminiscence to improve the wellbeing of those being cared for, to strengthen resilience to stress for carers, to enhance confidence and employability in the role, and to create productive relationships between those who care and those who are cared for, thereby improving the quality of care and the wellbeing of both. Further details can be obtained by emailing lisa.shaw@liverpool.ac.uk.

We are also developing different versions of the toolkit, initially one that includes film footage of Manchester in the 1960s–1970s, and we hope to expand the geographical coverage much further in due course. Lisa is continuing to expand her work in Brazil and is about to train a group of carers, as well as museum workers, at the Museum of Image and Sound in the city of Campinas, São Paulo state, in how they can use the Portuguese-language version of the toolkit and incorporate additional audio-visual material that is in plentiful supply in this museum and many others across the country, drawing on the rich national tradition of music listening and music-making, as well as the popularity of local films and their stars from the 'golden age' of the 1950s. Expanding our overseas collaborations, Lisa, Sara and Jacky are also developing a research project with partners in Chile, building on a pilot project currently underway in Liverpool that is exploring how the University of Liverpool's Popular Music Archive can help reconnect local people who came to Merseyside as exiles from the Chilean dictatorship of the 1970s–1980s reconnect with their past, form closer bonds with their younger family members and improve their wellbeing. They plan to take this idea to Chile and work with older people, including those living with a dementia diagnosis, to see how music can connect them to their younger selves in a positive way and enhance intergenerational bonds and understanding within families.

One area that we intend to develop in particular is precisely this bringing together of the younger and older generations, not only within families but in the wider community, to stimulate mutual wellbeing benefits via reminiscence and expressions of selfhood fostered by music and film. We are also keen to pursue the involvement of the 'users' of or participants in our future interventions and initiatives in their co-curation or co-production of workshops and events, thereby maximizing the wellbeing benefits by boosting a sense of agency, creativity and purpose. To this end, we will be seeking to work closely in partnership with cultural institutions and archives in the UK and Latin America in particular. Ultimately, our dream is to produce copies of the *Cinema,*

Memory and Wellbeing toolkit in a range of languages, drawing on audio-visual material tailored to the country in question, and to pilot these with a range of groups. As we work towards this goal, in the context of a wider large-scale, international and interdisciplinary research project, we will naturally be building on the findings and conclusions presented in this book, and for this depend on feedback from those of you who go on to download the toolkit and pilot its use in your own care context in the near future. We hope you enjoy using the toolkit and look forward to receiving your comments, observations and photographs.

AFTERWORD

Ros Jennings

In preparing the 'afterword' to this impressive publication I have had cause to reflect on my own journey from care assistant working with older people to my current role as an academic and Professor of Ageing, Culture and Media in a UK university. Considering the content of the book, it is not surprising that I was prompted to reflect on this journey. It is, however, testament to the power of this book that its 'affect' touches the intersectionalities of my journey so deeply. This is a book that addresses and engages with thinking, practices and most importantly people and their vulnerabilities. As such it is groundbreaking, and its impact will be internationally far-reaching in the formulation of approaches and therapeutic interventions to dementia care.

The authors collectively produce findings and reflections that engage authentically with the practices and experiences of doing academic work that aims to enhance the lives of the participants involved (both old people and also their carers). This work explores how, over the life course, popular films and music weave their way into the formation and production of memories and identities, and thus engage with individuals and groups via the past when the here and now has become confusing. Moreover, it explains how the intersections of the everyday and academic knowledge can be drawn on through multi-disciplinary methods of reminiscence to engage with people living with dementia and older people in care settings in the UK and Brazil. One of the achievements of the approaches trialed in this book is that benefits are also articulated by those who care for these people. Most importantly, the authors do not shy away from the difficulties and complexities involved in measuring, understanding and enhancing feelings of wellbeing in those involved in the studies. The self-reflexivity of the authors is crucial when faced with ethical questions around potential distress and differing perceptions about expressing emotions (especially when tears are shed).

The book offers a comprehensive and refreshing take on methods of engagement and some of the potential practical outcomes for academic researchers, professional carers and older people themselves. The concept of popular film and music as 'social prescription' is approached with caution and is not viewed as a potential panacea for the delivery of wellbeing to older people and those living with dementia. Instead the authors seek to apply their academic research on these media to address real-world needs and to improve and expand the resources available to promote high-quality care. The result is a set of findings and reflections that are refreshingly candid and accessible to academics and practitioners alike. The accompanying downloadable toolkit provides a platform for the sensitive implementation of creative methods in reminiscence activities that can be rolled out in a cost-effective way in care centres for the benefit of both participants and carers. This toolkit and book present a model that will be easily tailored to the specificities of other national contexts across the globe in due course.

Appendix

CINEMA, MEMORY AND WELLBEING QUESTIONNAIRES

<u>Cinema, Memory and Wellbeing (1st questionnaire)</u>

Name: Date:

Thank you for participating in the Cinema, Memory and Wellbeing project

Please indicate with a line through the scale 1...100

1. Overall how satisfied are you with your life nowadays?
   I am satisfied with my life just now
   0 = totally disagree 100 = totally agree

   0 ——————————————————100

2. Overall, to what extent do you feel the things you do in your life make you happy?
   My life has been happy so far.
   0 = totally disagree 100 = totally agree

   0 ——————————————————100

3. Overall how happy did you feel yesterday?
   I feel happy just now
   0 = totally disagree 100 = totally agree

   0 ——————————————————100

4. Overall how anxious did you feel yesterday?
   I feel anxious just now
   0 = totally disagree 100 = totally agree

   0 ——————————————————100

Cinema, Memory and Wellbeing (2nd questionnaire)

Name: Date:

Please answer the following questions just after seeing the film clips

Please indicate with a line through the scale 1...100

1. Overall how satisfied are you with your life nowadays?
    I am satisfied with my life just now
    0 = totally disagree 100 = totally agree

    0 ——————————————————————100

2. Overall, to what extent do you feel the things you do in your life make you happy?
    My life has been happy so far.
    0 = totally disagree 100 = totally agree

    0 ——————————————————————100

3. Overall how happy did you feel yesterday?
    I feel happy just now
    0 = totally disagree 100 = totally agree

    0 ——————————————————————100

4. Overall how anxious did you feel yesterday?
    I feel anxious just now
    0 = totally disagree 100 = totally agree

    0 ——————————————————————100

THANK YOU VERY MUCH

The following questions are about whether the films you have just seen made you think about your past and, if they did, what these memories were like for you. We'd like you to circle one of the three responses shown beneath each of the five questions to tell us about this please.

1. The films made me remember things about my life that I don't usually remember.

YES – DEFINITELY   YES – A BIT   NO – NOT REALLY

2. The films about Liverpool made me think about happy times.

YES – DEFINITELY   YES – A BIT   NO – NOT REALLY

3. The films about Liverpool made me think about less happy times.

YES – DEFINITELY   YES – A BIT   NO – NOT REALLY

4. The films with Carmen Miranda made me think about happy times.

YES – DEFINITELY   YES – A BIT   NO – NOT REALLY

5. The films with Carmen Miranda made me think about less happy times.

YES – DEFINITELY   YES – A BIT   NO – NOT REALLY

THANK YOU VERY MUCH

Cinema, Memory and Wellbeing (3rd questionnaire)

Name: Date:

Please answer the following questions the day after seeing the film clips

Please indicate with a line through the scale 1...100

1. Overall how satisfied are you with your life nowadays?
    I am satisfied with my life just now
    0 = totally disagree 100 = totally agree

    0 ————————————————————————100

2. Overall, to what extent do you feel the things you do in your life make you happy?
    My life has been happy so far.
    0 = totally disagree 100 = totally agree

    0 ————————————————————————100

3. Overall how happy did you feel yesterday?
    I feel happy just now
    0 = totally disagree 100 = totally agree

    0 ————————————————————————100

4. Overall how anxious did you feel yesterday?
    I feel anxious just now
    0 = totally disagree 100 = totally agree

    0 ————————————————————————100

THANK YOU VERY MUCH

REFERENCES

Atkinson, S., Bagnall, A. M., Corcoran, R., South, J., & Curtis, S. (2019). Being well together: Individual subjective and community wellbeing. *Journal of Happiness Studies*, 1–19. doi:10.1007/s10902-019-00146-2

Bamford, A., & Clift, S. (2007, January). *Making singing for health happen: Reflections on a "Singing for the Brain" training course.* Sidney De Hann Reports 2, Sidney De Haan Research Centre for Arts and Health, Folkestone.

Barrett, F. S., Grimm, K. J., Janata, P., Robins, R., Sedikides, C., & Wildschut, D. T. (2010). Music-evoked nostalgia: Affect, memory, and personality. *Emotion, 10*(3), 390–403.

Beerens, H. C., Sutcliffe, C., Renom-Guiteras, M., Soto, M. E., Suhonen, R., Zabalegui, A., … RightTimePlaceCare Consortium. (2014). Quality of life and quality of care for people with dementia receiving long term institutional care or professional home care: The European RightTimePlaceCare study. *Journal of the American Medical Directors Association, 15*(1), 54–61.

Bennett, A. (2013). *Music, style, and aging: Growing old disgracefully?* Philadelphia, PA: Temple University Press.

Bennett, A., & Rogers, I. (2016). Popular music and materiality: Memorabilia and memory traces. *Popular Music and Society*, *39*(1), 28–42.

Bergfelder, T., Shaw, L., & Vieira, J. L. (Eds.). (2017). *Stars and stardom in Brazilian cinema*. London and New York, NY: Palgrave Macmillan.

Parliament of the United Kingdom. (2014). Care Act. Retrieved from www.legislation.gov.uk. Accessed on June 2019.

Castillo, M. G., Ahmadi-Abhari, S., Bandosz, P., Capewell, S., Steptoe, A., Singh-Manoux, A., ... O'Flaherty, M. (2017). Forecasted trends in disability and life expectancy in England and Wales up to 2025: A modelling study. *Lancet Public Health*, *2*, 307–313.

CentreForum. (2014). The pursuit of happiness: A new ambition for our mental health. Retrieved from https://www.basw.co.uk/system/files/resources/basw_32003-1_0.pdf. Accessed on October 13, 2019.

Chao, S.-Y., Liu, H.-Y., Wu, C.-Y., Jin, S.-F., Chu, T.-L., Huang, T.-S., & Clark, M. (2006). The effects of group reminiscence therapy on depression, self esteem, and life satisfaction of elderly nursing home residents. *Journal of Nursing Research*, *14*, 36–45. doi:10.1097/01.JNR.0000387560.03823.c7

Chaudhury, H. (1999). Self and reminiscence of place: A conceptual study. *Journal of Aging and Identity*, *4*, 231–253. doi:10.1023/A:1022835109862

Cohen, S. (2014). "Going to a Gig": Remembering and mapping the places and journeys of live rock music in England. In K. Burland & S. Pitts (Eds.), *Coughing and clapping* (pp. 131–147). Farnham: Ashgate Publishing.

Cohen, S. (2016). Music as cartography: English audiences and their autobiographical memories of the musical past. In J. Brusila, B. Johnson, & J. Richardson (Eds.), *Music, memory, space* (pp. 107–123). Bristol: Intellect Books.

Cohen, S., & Kronenburg, R. (2018). *Musical landscapes: Liverpool.* London: Historic England.

Costa, F., Ockelford, A., & Hargreaves, D. J. (2018). Does regular listening to preferred music have a beneficial effect on symptoms of depression and anxiety amongst older people in residential care? The qualitative findings of a mixed methods study. *Music and Medicine: An Interdisciplinary Journal,* *10*(2), 54–62.

Cuddy, L. L., & Duffin, J. (2005). Music, memory, and Alzheimer's disease: Is music recognition spared in dementia, and how can it be assessed? *Medical Hypotheses, 64*(2), 229–235.

Dennison, S., & Shaw, L. (2004). *Popular cinema in Brazil, 1930–2001.* Manchester: Manchester University Press.

van Dijck, J. (2006). Record and hold: Popular music between personal and collective memory. *Critical Studies in Media Communication, 25*(5), 357–274.

Elias, S. M., Neville, C., & Scott, T. (2015). The effectiveness of group reminiscence therapy for loneliness, anxiety and depression in older adults in long-term care: A systematic review. *Geriatric Nursing, 36*(5), 372–380.

Engedal, K., & Laks, J. (2016). Towards a Brazilian dementia plan? Lessons to be learned from Europe. *Dementia & Neuropsychologica, 10*(2), 74–78.

Fancourt, D., Ockelford, A., & Belai, A. (2014). The psychoneuroimmunological effects of music: A systematic review and a new model. *Brain, Behavior, and Immunity, 36*, 15–26.

Foster, N. A., & Valentine, E. R. (1998). The effect of concurrent music on autobiographical recall in dementia clients. *Musicae Scientiae, 2*(2), 143–155.

Frith, S. (1996). Music and identity. In S. Hall & P. du Gay (Eds.), *Questions of cultural identity* (pp. 108–127). London: Sage Publications.

Gaggioli, A., Scaratti, C., Morganti, L., Stramba-Badiale, M., Agostoni, M., Spatola, C. A., … Riva, G. (2014). Effectiveness of group reminiscence for improving wellbeing of institutionalized elderly adults: Study protocol for a randomized controlled trial. *Trials, 15*, 408. doi:10.1186/1745-6215-15-408

Gallagher, M. (2017). A literature-based intervention for older people living with dementia. Retrieved from https://www.thereader.org.uk/literature-based-intervention-older-people-living-dementia/. Accessed on October 13, 2019.

Gallotti, M., & Frith, C. D. (2013). Social cognition in the we-mode. *Trends in Cognitive Sciences, 17*(4), 160–165.

Garcez-Lemme, L., & Deckers Lemme, M. (2014). Costs of elderly health care in Brazil: Challenges and strategies. *Medical Express, 1*(1). Retrieved from http://www.scielo.br/scielo.php?script=sci_arttext&pid=S2358-04292014000100003&lng=en&nrm=iso

Giebel, C. M., Sutcliffe, C., Stolt, M., Karlsson, S., Renom-Guiteras, A., Soto, M., … Challis, D. (2014). Deterioration of basic activities of daily living and their impact on quality of life across different cognitive stages of dementia: A

European study. *International Psychogeriatrics*, *26*(8), 1283–1293.

Gray, K., Evans, S. C., Griffiths, A., & Schneider, J. (2017). Critical reflections on methodological challenge in arts and dementia evaluation and research. *Dementia*, *17*(6), 775–784.

Hallam, J. (2005, 2nd ed. 2017). Remembering butterflies: The comic art of housework. In S. Lacey & J. Bignell (Eds.), *Popular television drama: New perspectives* (pp. 34–50). Manchester: Manchester University Press.

Hampson, C., & Morris, K. (2016). Dementia: Sustaining self in the face of cognitive decline. *Geriatrics*, *1*(25), 1–6.

Hays, T., & Minichiello, V. (2005). The meaning of music in the lives of older people: A qualitative study. *Psychology of Music*, *33*(4), 437–451.

Hsu, Y., & Wang, J. (2009). Physical, affective, and behavioral effects of group reminiscence on depressed institutionalized elders in Taiwan. *Nursing Research*, *58*(4), 294–299.

Houston, D. M., McKee, K. J., Carroll, L., & Marsh, H. (1998). Using humour to promote psychological wellbeing in residential homes for older people. *Aging and Mental Health*, *2*(4), 328–332.

Istvandity, L. (2017). Combining music and reminiscence therapy interventions for well-being in elderly populations: A systematic review. *Complementary Therapies in Clinical Practice*, *28*, 18–25.

Jacobsen, J. H., Stelzer, J., Fritz, T. H., Chételat, G., La Joie, R., & Turner, R. (2015). Why musical memory can be preserved in advanced Alzheimer's disease. *Brain*, *138*(8), 2438–2450.

Johnson, R., & Taylor, C. (2011). Can playing pre-recorded music at mealtimes reduce the symptoms of agitation for people with dementia? *International Journal of Therapy and Rehabilitation, 18*(12), 700–708.

Keightley, K. (1996). "Turn it down!" She shrieked: Gender, domestic space, and high fidelity, 1948–59. *Popular Music, 15*(2), 149–177.

Kindell, J., Burrow, S., Wilkinson, R., & David Keady, J. (2014). Life story resources in dementia care: A review. *Quality in Ageing and Older Adults, 15*(3), 151–161. doi: 10.1108/QAOA-02-2014-0003

Kitwood, T., & Bredin, K. (1992). Towards a theory of dementia care: Personhood and well-being. *Ageing and Society, 12*(3), 269–287.

Kuhn, A. (1995). *Family secrets: Acts of memory and imagination*. London and New York, NY: Verso.

Kuhn, A. (2002). *An everyday magic: Cinema and cultural memory*. London and New York, NY: I. B. Tauris.

Kuhn, A. (2010). Memory texts and memory work: Performances of memory in and with visual media. *Memory Studies, 3*(4), 298–313.

Latha, K. S., Bhandary, P. V., Tejaswini, S., & Sahana, M. (2014). Reminiscence therapy: An overview. *Middle East Journal of Age and Ageing, 11*(1). doi:10.5742/MEAA. 2014.92393

Lewis, C. N. (1971). Reminiscing and self-concept in old age. *Journal of Gerontology, 26*(2), 240–243.

MacDonald, R., Kreutz, G., & Mitchell, L. (2012). What is music, health, and wellbeing and why is it important?

In R. MacDonald, G. Kreutz, & L. Mitchell (Eds.),
Music, health and wellbeing. Oxford: Oxford University Press.

MacDonald, R., Miell, D., & Wilson, G. (2005). Talking about
music: A vehicle for identity development. In D. Miell, R.
MacDonald, & D. J. Hargreaves (Eds.), *Musical communication*
(pp. 321–338). Oxford: Oxford University Press.

Mosby's medical dictionary (8th ed.). (2009). Edinburgh,
London and Amsterdam: Elsevier.

O'Connor, D., Phinney, A., Smith, A., Small, J., Purves, B.,
Perry, J., … Beattie, L. (2007). Personhood in dementia care:
Developing a research agenda for broadening the vision.
Dementia, 6, 121–142.

Osman, S., Tischler, V., & Schneider, J. (2016). Singing for
the brain: A qualitative study exploring the health and
wellbeing benefits of singing for people with dementia and
their carers. *Dementia*, *15*(6), 1326–1339.

Patterson, M. C., & Perlstein, S. (2011). Good for the heart,
good for the soul: The creative arts and brain health in later
life. *Generations – Journal of the American Society on Aging*,
35(2), 27–36.

Pickering, M., & Keightley, E. (2015). *Photography, music
and memory: Pieces of the past in everyday life*. London:
Palgrave Macmillan.

Platz, F., Kopiez, R., Hasselhorn, J., & Wolf, A. (2015). The
impact of song-specific age and affective qualities of popular
songs on music-evoked autobiographical memories
(MEAMs). *Musicae Scientiae*, *19*(4), 327–349.

Rathbone, C. J., Moulin, C. J., & Conway, M. A. (2008). Self-
centered memories: The reminiscence bump and self. *Memory
and Cognition*, *36*(8), 1403–1414.

Satorres, E., Viguer, P., Fortunam, F. B., & Meléndez, J. C. (2017). Effectiveness of instrumental reminiscence intervention on improving coping in healthy older adults. *Stress and Health: Journal of the International Society for the Investigation of Stress*, 34(2), 227–234.

Shaw, L. (2013). *Carmen Miranda*. London: Palgrave Macmillan/BFI.

Shaw, L., & Dennison, S. (2007). *Brazilian National Cinema*. London: Routledge.

Stacey, J. (1993). *Star Gazing: Hollywood cinema and female spectatorship*. London: Routledge.

Surr, C. A. (2006). Preservation of self in people with dementia living in residential care: A socio-biographical approach. *Social Science and Medicine*, 62(7), 1720–1730.

Tamura-Lis, W. (2017). Reminiscing – A tool for excellent elder care and improved quality of life. *Urologic Nursing*, 37(3), 151–156.

The Kings Fund. (2017). What is social prescribing? Retrieved from https://www.kingsfund.org.uk/publications/social-prescribing?gclid=EAIaIQobChMI7fjJpLit5QIVQUTTCh0dRAJ2EAAYASAAEgIBVfD_BwE. Accessed on October 20, 2019.

Therrien, A. (2018). Daily chats improve lives of people with dementia. *BBC News*, February 7. Retrieved from https://www.bbc.co.uk/news/health-42918345. Accessed on October 13, 2019.

Touhy, T. A., & Jett, K. F. (2016). Communicating with older adults. In T. A. Touhy & K. F. Jett (Eds.), *Ebersole & Hess' toward healthy aging: Human needs & nursing response* (pp. 65–73). St. Louis, MO: Elsevier/Mosby.

Tse, M., Lo, A. P., Cheng, T. L., Chan, E. K., Chan, A. H., & Chung, H. S. (2010). Humor therapy: Relieving chronic pain and enhancing happiness for older adults. *Journal of Aging Research*, 9 pp., Article ID 343574. doi:10.4061/2010/343574

Verbeek, H., Meyer, G., Challis, D., Zabalegui, A., Soto, M. E., Saks, K., … RightTimePlaceCare Consortium. (2015). Inter-country exploration of factors associated with admission to long-term institutional dementia care: Evidence from the RightTimePlaceCare study. *Journal of Advanced Nursing*, 71(6), 1338–1350.

Verbeek, H., Meyer, G., Leino-Kilpi, H., Zabalegui, A., Hallberg, I. R., Saks, K., … RightTimePlaceCare Consortium. (2012). A European study investigating patterns of transition from home care towards institutional dementia care: The protocol of a RightTimePlaceCare study. *BMC Public Health*, 12(68). Retrieved from https://link.springer.com/article/10.1186/1471-2458-12-68

Windle, G., Algar-Skaife, K., Caulfield, M., Pickering-Jones, L., Killick, J., Zeilig, H., & Tischler, V. (2019, March). Enhancing communication between dementia care staff and their residents: An arts-inspired intervention. *Aging and Mental Health*, 1–10. Retrieved from https://www.tandfonline.com/doi/full/10.1080/13607863.2019.1590310

Yates, S., & Lockely, E. (2018). Social media and social class. *American Behavioral Scientist*, 62(9), 1291–1316.

Young, R., Camic, P. M., & Tischler, V. (2016). The impact of community-based arts and health interventions on cognition in people with dementia: A systematic literature review. *Aging and Mental Health*, 20(4), 337–351.

FILMS AND TELEVISION PROGRAMMES

Alive Inside (Rossato-Bennett, 2014).

Down Argentine Way (Irving Cummings, 1940).

É de chuá! (Victor Lima, 1958).

Our Dementia Choir with Vicky McClure (BBC, 2019).

The Gangs All Here (Busby Berkeley, 1943).

The Magnet (Charles Frend, 1950).

That Night in Rio (Irving Cummings, 1941).

Um Candango na Belacap (Roberto Farias, 1961).

Violent Playground (Basil Dearden, 1958).

INDEX

Printed in the United States
By Bookmasters